THE 10 POUNDS OFF PALEO DIET

From the experts at Cooking Light

THE 10 POUNDS OFF PALEO DIET

The Easy Way to Drop Inches in Just 28 Days

Oxmoor House®

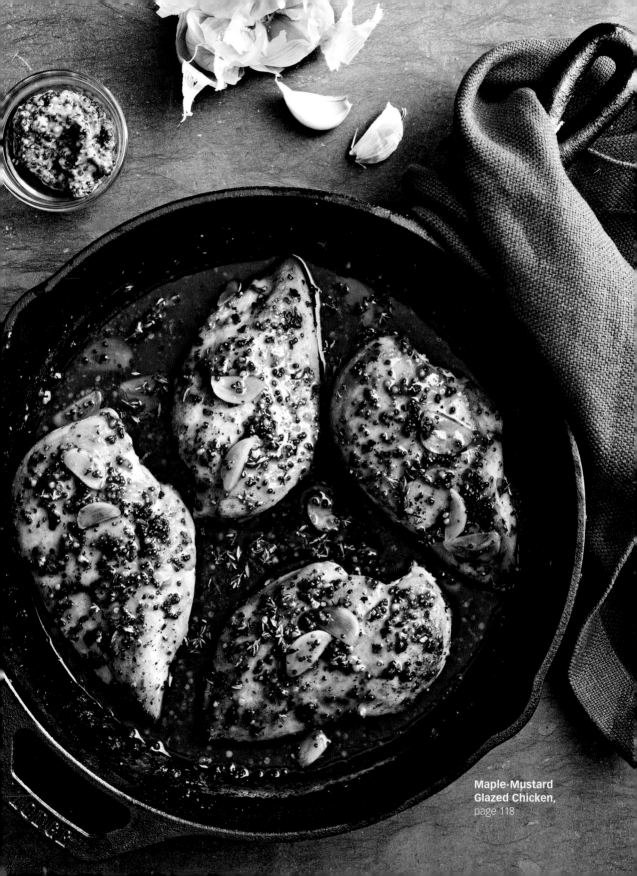

Maple-Mustard
Glazed Chicken,
page 118

CONTENTS

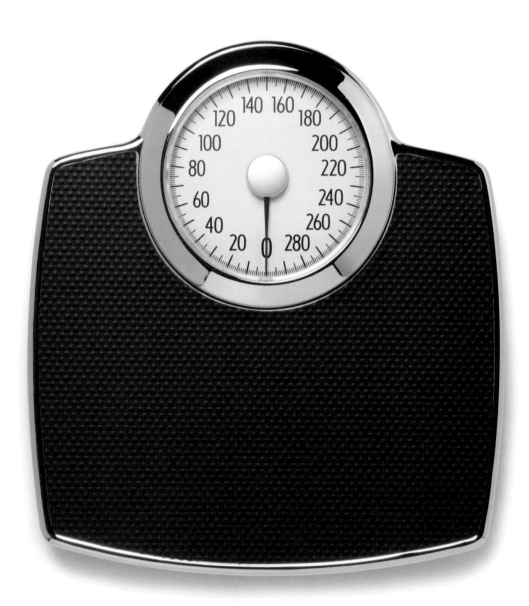

WHO DOESN'T WANT TO SEE THE SCALE 10 POUNDS LIGHTER? This book will show you how to do just that while adhering to a Paleo eating plan. In the following pages, you'll find a comprehensive introduction to the diet (complete with cutting-edge research) as well as 100 recipes from the healthy cooking experts at *Cooking Light*, four weeks of meal plans, and a do-anywhere fitness plan to help you tone up and slim down—safely, easily, and deliciously.

PART 1

PALEO
POWER

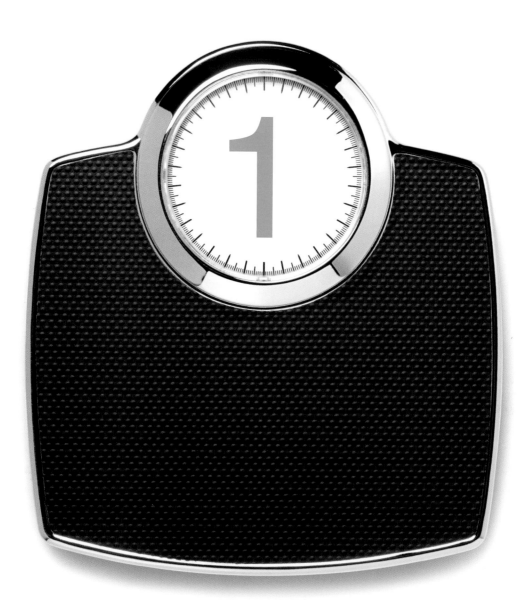

YOU'VE NO DOUBT HEARD A LOT ABOUT THE PALEOLITHIC DIET. Maybe you know it as the Caveman Diet or *Stone Age Diet*—or just Paleo. Friends may have tried it. You might have read about its aversion to grains and cut back on gluten with the idea that it might help you shed a few pounds. Maybe you've tried to avoid processed foods or decided to eat more raw stuff.

The diet may sound simple at first, but it's actually based on a relatively complex idea. The concept was first proposed at length in a self-published book called *The Stone Age Diet,* by Walter L. Voegtlin, M.D. A gastroenterologist, Voegtlin based his theory of the ideal diet on the way the human body was built and anthropological research. He came to the conclusion that we evolved primarily to eat a protein-based diet, one that focused on meat and other foods readily at hand that were eaten raw or with basic preparation.

Voegtlin gained some notoriety for his revolutionary ideas, but the diet didn't really start to gain attention until 1985, when two doctors, Boyd Eaton and Melvin Konner, expanded on Voegtlin's theories in a *New England Journal of Medicine* paper called "Paleolithic Nutrition." The basic concept was that we have spent around 200,000 years in a hunter-gatherer state, and as a result, we've evolved to eat a certain way. Our bodies thrive and in fact depend on basic nutritional principles that we've lost touch with over the millennia. Since we haven't evolved much in the last 10,000 years—about when we began farming—our bodies and digestive systems are still best suited to the diet our Paleolithic ancestors consumed.

One of the more interesting findings over the past several decades is that our ancient forebears actually lived longer and healthier lives than anthropologists once thought. Paleolithic men and women were about as tall as we are now, they lived about as long, and the remains that anthropologists have analyzed suggest our ancestors had little experience with the health concerns so common in the modern world, such as heart disease, diabetes, and cancer.

The diet our Paleolithic forebears ate would be one we're uniquely suited to consume. So what exactly is it? After poring over the findings of anthropologists, Eaton, Konner, and others have concluded that we ate what we could capture—and this was the biggest caloric reward we could hope for. When we couldn't capture and kill our meals, we picked the edible nonprotein food sources around us: nuts,

TIP

Recruit a partner.
Getting your spouse, friend, or other family member to join you will help you get off to a good start. The two of you can share ideas, recipes, and keep each other on track through the tough times.

berries, fruit, and some roots. Because of food scarcity, survival depended on gleaning the highest caloric rewards from our food—and that's how we became efficient digesters. Our digestive tract is relatively short and simple compared to animals that are vegetarian.

Now, of course, we've lived a long time as harvesters of grains and agricultural growers, so it seems like our bodies would have adapted to these relatively new foodstuffs. Not so fast: Evolutionary scientists say that in fact our bodies have changed remarkably little in the last 10,000 years. And it's during that time that our problems with chronic diseases began to emerge.

Why Paleo Is The Perfect Plan

When you set out to shed just a few pounds—which is a great way to approach weight loss, whether you want to lose 10 or 100 pounds—the best thing to do is to keep your diet simple. A huge Paleo advantage is that you don't have to weigh food, elaborately plan meals, or count calories.

That may seem liberating—or maybe a little frightening, if you're used to diets with rigid rules. With Paleo, you don't have to count calories because eating the foods you're meant to consume will help you naturally feel full before you're at risk of overeating. You'll stay satisfied for much longer than when you eat the cheap, nutritionally unfulfilling foods so common in our modern diet. The other advantage is that eliminating foods the body struggles to digest and process will help reduce inflammation. Considering that being overweight and obese are primarily diseases of inflammation, taming the fire within the body will help you shed pounds even more quickly. You may find your initial weight loss far surpasses your 10-pound goal. Although dieting experts set the pace of safe weight loss at 2 pounds per week, soothing inflammation may mean that you lose even twice that much in the first several weeks.

TIP

Start slowly. If you love bread or pasta and can't imagine life without it, don't try going cold turkey or you'll be setting yourself up for failure. Instead, try limiting your grains to one meal a day, and then reduce the size of your grain serving before you eliminate it entirely.

Lose Belly Fat Faster

Carrying extra pounds around the midsection may be the most troubling aspect of being overweight. Research has found that too much belly fat is harder on organs, arteries, and the heart than fat you carry elsewhere, such as on your hips or thighs. According to new research, you may be able to target that spare tire if you fill your plate with the right foods.

At McMaster University in Ontario, researchers recruited 90 overweight and obese women and put them on a regular exercise schedule of walking and strength training. They also assigned them to one of three diets, featuring high, medium, and low amounts of protein. The researchers measured the volunteers' fat and muscle both at the beginning of the study and four months later, at the end. While all the women lost the same amount of weight on average, the big difference was in their levels of fat and muscle: 100 percent of the weight loss in the high-protein group was fat, especially around the midsection. They also added about a pound and a half of muscle, while the low-protein group actually lost 1.5 pounds of muscle. "The preservation or even gain of muscle is very important for maintaining metabolic rate and preventing weight regain, which can be a major problem for many seeking to lose weight," says Andrea Josse, lead author of the study and a graduate student in the Department of Kinesiology at McMaster.

How much protein did the women who had the most weight loss consume? The amounts weren't too daunting: They got about 30 percent of their calories from protein—about what you get on a Paleo plan; most Americans typically get in the neighborhood of 15 to 20 percent.

Shed Pounds

Everyone knows that eating fewer calories than you burn through exercise and daily activity can lead to weight loss. But one thing researchers have learned in the last decade is how the calories you eat influence appetite. The biggest surprise was that low-fiber carbohydrates—think of rice cakes, white-flour bread and crackers, low-fat high-sugar treats—could actually increase hunger. These easily digested carbohydrates are similar in structure to the blood sugar—glucose—that powers your body. The sudden surge of glucose provokes a rise in insulin, the hormone your body relies on to process sugar. All that glucose either gets burned up for energy or shuttled off to places like your thighs and belly to be converted to long-term storage—in other words, fat.

The rapid peak and then plunge in blood sugar is a source of weight-gain troubles. As levels fall, your gut signals your brain that energy supplies are running low, and then you're hungry again. The calories you consumed make you want to eat more, and suddenly the calories-in vs. calories-out equation doesn't add up the way we always thought it did.

The solution is to add more protein to your diet—fish, lean cuts of meat, and nuts are good choices. All these foods take longer to digest, resulting in a more gradual rise of blood sugar. You'll feel full longer and give yourself a chance to tip the scale in your favor.

You've probably heard about the all-meat Atkins plan. That's not the answer. You may be able to lose some weight by eating bacon, lamb, and steak morning, noon, and night, but you won't feel very good, and you'll be as likely to have long-term success on Atkins as you would a wheatgrass-and-kale diet. But when researchers scrutinized the high-protein approach of Atkins, they discovered something they didn't expect: People who ate higher-protein diets lost more weight than people on high-carbohydrate plans, but they were also far more likely to stay on the diet than the high-carb dieters. Even better, the protein eaters tended to preserve muscle and lose more fat compared to the high-carb group.

People who eat protein at breakfast—a poached egg, for example—eat 100 to 200 fewer calories the rest of the day than people who have toast and jam, low-fiber cereal, or other simple carbohydrate breakfasts. As you'll find, a

TIP

Just because you're eating more protein doesn't mean you can forget about produce. Make sure your house is stocked with plenty of healthy produce. Keep in-season fruit nearby, and store greens, mushrooms, squash, onions, and other Paleo-friendly produce in the crisper drawer of your fridge.

lunch of sliced turkey or chicken over a salad of greens allows you to make it to dinner with minimal snacking.

You may discover that as you start this diet you'll actually shed pounds much more quickly than the recommended average of 2 pounds a week. Don't worry about that—beginning a new plan will fill you with energy, and that may lead you to be more active, burn more calories, and shed weight faster. Plus, as inflammation levels fall, the pounds (and your water weight) will disappear. Within a week or two your face and shape will look noticeably different in the mirror!

The Health Benefits of Going Paleo

Health is one of the biggest concerns dieters have when adopting this plan. And in fact some researchers and diet experts still debate whether an approach that favors protein and eliminates whole grains can really claim to be safe. You'll be happy to hear that the trend in research is supporting the idea that an approach like Paleo may actually be healthier for you.

In a huge 2014 study from Boston University Medical Center that was published in the *American Journal of Hypertension,* researchers analyzed the diets and health of more than 5,000 individuals and then followed them for 11 years to see who would go on to develop high blood pressure. Their findings revealed that the more protein the study subjects regularly ate, the lower their blood pressure. The results held true even for people who were overweight—and being overweight by itself is a risk factor for high blood pressure. Remarkably, eating more protein reduced blood pressure by 40 to 60 percent in the study subjects. "These results provide no evidence to suggest that individuals concerned about the development of high blood pressure should avoid dietary protein," explains study author Lynn Moore, M.D., an associate professor of medicine at Boston University. "Rather, protein intake may play a role in the long-term prevention of high blood pressure."

"I never dreamed that living the Paleo lifestyle would have changed my life this much. I'm way more energetic now."

Success Story:
Sarah

Within one year of trying a Paleo diet, Sarah lost nearly 80 pounds. "At a whopping 273 pounds, my body was shutting down. Everything hurt, I couldn't breathe properly, and I was emotionally wrecked," she explains. "After I went Paleo, I found my immune system started working much better. Today, I rarely get sick."

Now, four years later, she's kept the weight off and she's passionate about helping others learn that it is possible to find weight loss success. Sarah encourages and educates others by working for a professional Paleo blogger.

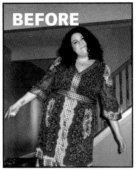

BEFORE

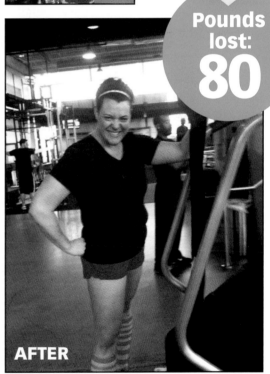

AFTER

Age: **33**

Height: **5'10"**

Weight before: **273**

Weight after: **193**

Pounds lost: **80**

Moore believes dietary guidelines need to be rewritten to emphasize the importance of protein in protecting the heart.

Weight-loss studies in general have been supporting the ideas behind Paleo. A 2014 study from Harvard Medical School found that over a year and a half, people who followed a high-protein plan had lower inflammation, cholesterol, and triglycerides—all of which are linked to a higher risk of heart disease. People who followed a more traditional low-fat diet actually got worse. Again, the take-home for the Paleo dieter is that not only is this diet more likely to help him/her lose weight, it seems to be healthier as well.

Researchers at the Johns Hopkins University School of Medicine kept a close watch on the arteries of 23 overweight and obese people as they followed a typical high-protein plan. Participants limited their carbohydrates to no more than 30 percent of their total calories, while they allowed fats from lean meat, dairy, and nuts to make up as much as 40 percent of their calories. Despite their diet's high-fat content (traditional diet advice is to limit fat to less than 30 percent of calories), it didn't alter key measurements of artery health, such as flexibility, the researchers found. What's more, compared to volunteers following a more traditional low-fat diet, the high-fat dieters lost weight much more quickly: They dropped 10 pounds in 45 days, while the low-fat group required a total of 70 days to lose the same.

"Our study should help allay the concerns that many people who need to lose weight have about choosing a low-carb diet instead of a low-fat one, and provide reassurance that both types of diet are effective at weight loss and that a low-carb approach does not seem to pose any immediate risk to vascular health," says the study's lead researcher, exercise physiologist Kerry Stewart, Ed.D. "More people should be considering a low-carb diet as a good option." If you're concerned about harming your heart with this plan, worry no more.

TIP

Before starting any diet, get a physical and check with your doctor about your health. Not only will you be radically changing your diet, but you'll also be exercising more, and you'll be more active in general thanks to your increased energy. For these reasons, you'll want to talk to your doctor about your plans.

Other Health Benefits to Paleo

Diabetes has reached epidemic numbers in the United States. According to the Centers for Disease Control and Prevention (CDC), between 1980 and 2011 the number of people with diabetes increased 133 percent. The source of this dramatic increase is weight related, no question. Diabetes incidence has marched in lockstep with the increase in people who are overweight and obese. But there's another culprit at work: inflammation.

You've already read about inflammation here and elsewhere, no doubt. It can result from low-grade chronic infections, pain, or stress. But perhaps simple carbs are the easiest source of inflammation to spot—and to control—in our diet. Eating so much sugar and other forms of carbohydrates day in and day out dramatically raises the level of inflammation in the body. Researchers call this phenomenon silent inflammation.

Gökhan Hotamisligil, M.D., Ph.D., professor of genetics and metabolism at the Harvard School of Public Health, is one of the leading researchers in the area of silent inflammation and how it relates to obesity. This silent inflammation spurs the steady release of pro-inflammatory chemicals into the blood, which can raise the risk of diabetes by interfering with insulin's ability to remove glucose from the bloodstream while increasing blood pressure by swelling arteries, which drives up heart-disease risk. Chronic inflammation has even been tied to dementia and cancer.

As Hotamisligil and others—including Barry Sears, Ph.D., founder of the Inflammation Research Foundation and author of *The Zone*—looked more closely at this inflammation, they discovered it can promote weight gain by suppressing hormones that help control appetite and blood sugar. The result: You lose a sense of how full you are, and your blood sugar soars and plunges, triggering the impulse to eat more.

What Sears and other researchers have found is that many of the most popular types of food we eat support and enhance this inflammatory state in the body. Carbohydrates are the main source, but there are other culprits. You may have heard of omega-3 fatty acids, the healthy fats found in fish and nuts. One of the reasons omega-3s bestow health benefits is that they're anti-inflammatory. However, this healthy fat has a brother called omega-6, and it's far more common in our food supply. We get it from vegetable oils such as corn, soy, and safflower—oils that have been promoted as healthy, but new research demonstrates they are in fact inflammatory. Our bodies also convert refined carbohydrate-rich foods—pastries, white bread, and fructose sweeteners in soda—into omega-6. The fat isn't really that bad, says Sears, but it needs to be in balance with omega-3s in our diet or it will spur inflammation. The problem is that omega-6 foods are the cheapest form of calories in our diet and are widely used in the manufacture of most processed foods—a practice that began in the 1970s around the time Americans began to develop a weight problem.

Another inflammation-related disease is polycystic ovary syndrome (PCOS), a hormonal imbalance that can lead to distressing symptoms, including weight gain and obesity—as many as one in five women battle this condition. New research from the University of Copenhagen in Denmark has found that a diet that favors healthy sources of protein over carbohydrates can help women with PCOS manage symptoms and lose weight. Scientists recruited 57 women with PCOS to take part in the study. Half the women followed a traditional diet that got about 15 percent of its calories from protein, 55 percent from carbs, and 30 percent from fat. The rest followed a high-protein plan—more than 40 percent of calories from protein and less than 30 percent of calories from carbs, with the last 30 percent coming from fat. After six months, the researchers discovered that women on the high-protein plan lost more than twice the weight of those on the high-carb plan—17 pounds versus 7 pounds. And a much higher percentage of the loss was in the form of fatty tissue: The protein eaters shed 14 pounds of fat compared to the 5 pounds lost by the carb group.

Weight loss alone can help lessen the symptoms of PCOS, say the researchers. The protein group also experienced healthy improvements in hormones and blood sugar control compared to the carb group. Researchers say that it's clear eating more healthy protein—red meat, turkey, chicken, and dairy—can help women with this condition.

Again and again, research demonstrates that the best way to balance your diet and reduce inflammation is to add healthy protein to your diet and shed pounds. Sears and Hotamisligil have found that losing even a few pounds can dramatically lower markers of inflammation in the blood. (Reducing stress will also help, and exercise is a great way to manage life's stressors. You can get more bang for your buck by ensuring your exercise is relaxing—yoga can fit the bill—but you'll learn more about that later.)

The step that everyone should take is to avoid pro-inflammatory foods and seek out anti-inflammatory meals, and the best way to do that is to adopt a Paleo approach to eating!

We've Come a Long Way

Just 10 years ago, government health experts and most major health organizations recommended a low-fat diet with no more than 30 percent of your calories from fat. Then studies at Harvard and elsewhere revealed that people following low-fat diets were more likely to abandon their diets compared to people who followed regimens that contained as much as 40 percent of calories from fat.

What's more, there's no evidence that low-fat vegetarian or vegan diets produce more weight loss than a plan that features plenty of healthy fats like those in olive oil, fatty fish, and coconuts. Animal and plant proteins contain anti-inflammatory substances; in the following chapters you'll read more about how pastured, traditionally raised meats such as free-range chickens (and eggs) and grass-fed red meat will deliver the omega-3 fats your diet is missing. And you don't have to worry about the saturated fat content from eggs, beef, and coconut oil: Once considered damaging to your heart, saturated fat got a reprieve when investigators found some types of saturated fatty acids may not have a negative effect on cholesterol. But the biggest reason to go Paleo and add these healthy fat-containing foods to your diet is that it simply tastes better. The possible health benefits are just a bonus.

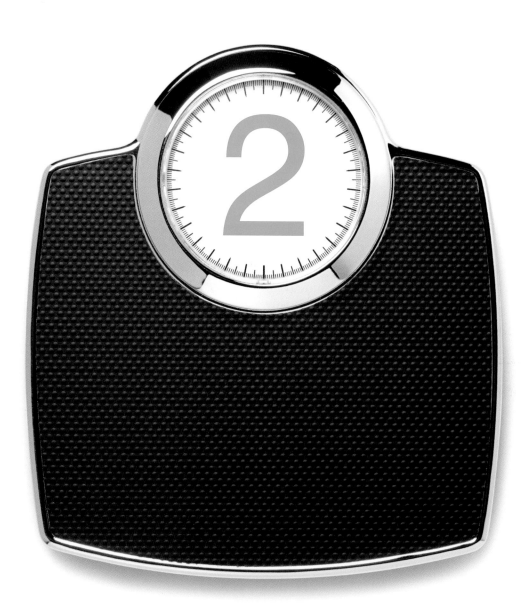

WHY GOING PALEO IS GOOD FOR YOU

THE ZONE. ATKINS. DUKAN. All of these diets promote a high-protein approach. Each plan comes with promises of dramatic weight loss. And all of them fall short of Paleo in one fashion or another. Part of the problem with these plans is that they don't take into account the quality of the food you eat or the true biology of your body.

Probably the biggest difference between the foods allowed on the Paleo diet as compared to other high-protein, low-carb diets is the type of carbohydrate and protein recommended. Basically, if our hunter-gatherer ancestors didn't have access to the food, then it isn't Paleo-friendly.

No Processed Food

As researchers probe the modern diet to find out what went wrong—why does modern food cause people to blow up like balloons?—they've repeatedly come back to one fundamental truth: Processed food, which is factory produced; packed with salt, sugar, and artificial flavorings; and stripped of vital nutrients, equals disaster for the body. Despite the obvious downside of these frankenfoods, most high-protein plans allow you to fill your daily diet with them. Some plans even produce their own processed meals for sale in your local grocery store.

The issue with these low-quality foodstuffs is that while they may temporarily fill you up, they actually leave your body starving for good nutrition. You feel hungry after a big meal because you're craving the missing vitamins and minerals, not to mention the phytonutrients, antioxidants, and other valuable disease-fighting substances in unprocessed foods.

Fast food falls into this category as well: You wouldn't believe how many chemicals and flavorings are pumped into the average burger from a fast food chain. The sodium and sugar contents in the food you get is astronomically high: This stuff has been tested and tinkered with for decades to arrive at a food that is designed to trigger extreme taste sensations that will keep you coming back. By cutting fast food out of your diet, you'll rediscover the true, satisfying, and pleasurable flavors of real food.

Plenty of Produce

Another difference between Paleo and high-protein plans is that Paleo isn't really low carbohydrate. Most high-protein diets restrict carb intake to about 25 percent or less of your total calories. They manage to do this by limiting the consumption of healthy fruits and vegetables.

That approach deprives you of valuable disease-fighting substances that can also help you lose weight. And it really doesn't make any sense from an evolutionary standpoint. Think about our cavemen ancestors—the ones responsible for our genetic makeup and digestive system: Would they pass up a bush of ripe blackberries? Turn their nose up at wild mangoes? Avoid apples, peppers, tomatoes, or any other wild produce they stumbled upon?

Not a chance. Cavemen sought out food wherever they could find it, and if that meant foraging for fruits and vegetables, that was much easier and less dangerous than trying to bring down a wild animal. On this Paleo diet, you'll get up to 40 percent of your calories from carbohydrates in the form of the natural starches and sugars contained in fresh produce.

Good-bye Grains

Perhaps the primary distinction between Paleo and other high-protein diets is that on Paleo, you'll eliminate cereal grains like wheat, corn, barley, and rye. While that may give you pause, there are actually several compelling reasons to get grains out of your diet—primarily because our digestive tracts aren't really set up to deal with them. Evolutionarily speaking, farming practices are relatively new to humans, and our guts aren't set up to effectively digest grains. But you might be surprised to hear that over the last 100 years, farming practices have altered grains and they've become even more harmful and difficult to digest. Here are some of the problems eating wheat and other grains can cause:

• **Inflamed gut**: A component of wheat, barley, and rye—gluten— creates trouble for many people. Grains have been selectively bred to contain more gluten; food scientists believe that nowadays, wheat contains nearly 10 times the amount of gluten it did 50 years ago. Gluten is a protein that can prompt an autoimmune reaction in the gut. Your own immune system attacks the digestive tract, which interferes with digestion and can lead to malnutrition, irritable bowel syndrome, or in some cases weight gain, finds researchers at the University of Chicago. The World Health Organization reports that as many 1 in 100 people have an inherited chronic form of gluten sensitivity known as celiac disease; an additional one-third of the general population may be suffering from inflammation caused by a reaction to gluten.

• **Increased hunger:** One of the challenges when dieting is recognizing when you're full. A form of protein in wheat called lectin actually short-circuits communication between your stomach and your brain: This protein binds with hunger receptors in your intestine and blocks the signals your gut sends when it's full.

• **Hormonal overload:** One of the problems of our modern lifestyle is that we're exposed to too many hormones—especially xenoestrogens, which are chemicals that mimic the female hormone estrogen and promote the retention of fat. One way we're exposed to these xenoestrogens is through grains, thanks to the pesticides, herbicides, and fungicides that factory farms use on crops. In women, this faux hormone can trigger the buildup of fat around the thighs, hips, and belly; in men, they swell the waistline and encourage gynecomastia—the swelling of breast tissue.

• **Sluggish thyroid:** To get soft pillowy slices of bread, food makers rely on a chemical dough conditioner called potassium bromate. The problem is this conditioner also happens to be an endocrine disruptor—it interrupts the flow of the body's natural hormones and has been linked to an increased risk of thyroid cancer. But long before it spurs tumor growth, the conditioner can slow down your thyroid. One of this gland's jobs is to regulate metabolism; as the gland's activity decreases, so does your metabolism. That equals fewer calories burned and more fat on your body.

• **Starchy surprise:** Food scientists call a critical ingredient in bread—amylopectin A—the super starch. This starch helps bread rise and become fluffy, but in your body it behaves just like white sugar: It dramatically raises blood sugar. That leads to inflammation and insulin resistance because your body must work extra hard to process all that sugar.

Why Paleo Is a Nutritionally Complete and Healthy Diet

A concern for people beginning a Paleo diet is whether they'll get the nutrients they need. The good news is that several studies have demonstrated that eating the full complement of Paleo foods does provide all the nutrients you need. Research by Loren Cordain, Ph.D., one of the originators of the Paleo diet, has found that eating this way can provide anywhere from double to 10 times the amount of your daily requirements for vitamins and minerals. There's no reason to take supplements with this diet.

You might be worried about your bones since you've eliminated a major source of calcium by cutting out dairy. But you more than make up for it with dark greens, fish, fruit, seeds, and nuts. Plus, you'll be getting more of the nutrients that help your body process calcium from your diet, such as magnesium, potassium, and vitamin K. As a result, you won't miss the calcium from dairy at all.

With the absence of grains in Paleo, you may think you'll need to scrounge up other sources of fiber. But you'll be eating many more fruits, vegetables, and seeds than you did previously, and these provide all the fiber your body requires.

Perhaps the biggest concern people have about Paleo is the amount of fat. One nutritional fact that's been drilled into our heads is that meat is bad and that too much of it will dangerously raise your intake of fats—especially the most dangerous fat of all, saturated.

Full disclosure: You will eat a lot more fat on a Paleo diet. But here's the good news: That fat will not only help you lose weight, it will help you avoid heart disease and weight-related illnesses.

How could this be? The best story to come out of nutrition research in the last several years is the one about how good fat can be for your body. It began when researchers realized that monounsaturated fats like those found in olives and avocados could reduce the risk of heart disease.

Then diet researchers at the Harvard School of Public Health found that people trying to lose weight were more successful when they ate more fat, not less. Then something really strange happened.

In 2011, some of the sharpest nutritional minds in the world met in Copenhagen, Denmark, to settle a nagging question: Is saturated fat really bad for you? The doctors traveled from Britain, France, The Netherlands, Sweden, Australia, and the United States. They hailed from respected institutions like the Institut Pasteur de Lille, King's College London, and the Harvard School of Public Health. For two days they batted around evidence on diet, reviewing 50 years' worth of studies. They looked at research done in petri dishes and on mice, monkeys, and humans.

You would think the answer is obvious based on what we've been told for the past 50 years, but it's not. The symposium's results, which were published in the *American Journal of Clinical Nutrition,* indicate that many saturated-fat containing foods aren't as dangerous as we thought. And they're considerably safer than the refined carbohydrate items we've replaced them with.

What happened? As it turns out, there have been rumblings for years that saturated fat may not be the ogre experts believed. In the early 2000s, several studies by researchers at Harvard and other institutions pitted low-fat, high-carbohydrate diets against high-protein (and higher-fat) diets. In study after study, weight loss was slightly better on the high-protein plans— a surprise for many diet experts. But more importantly, heart disease risk factors like high cholesterol and high blood pressure actually decreased when people ate more fat. That wasn't supposed to happen: Adding fat to the diet should have increased fat in the blood, which is responsible for clogging arteries and triggering heart trouble.

The discovery that diets featuring saturated fat could reduce heart risk factors led Ronald Krauss, M.D., director of heart disease research at the Children's Hospital Oakland Research Institute, to review earlier studies that had fingered saturated fat as the bad guy. Krauss and his colleagues found that people who replaced foods high in saturated fat with those containing refined carbohydrates failed to improve their overall risk of heart disease. In fact, their risk worsened. The original studies had focused on

> "Within just three weeks of following a Paleo diet, my fears of needing surgery for my lower GI issues were gone."

Success Story:
Bob

In 2006, Bob was 22 years old and working in the restaurant business in Atlantic City. He ate and drank whatever he wanted until his weight had climbed to 268 pounds. That's when Bob decided he needed to make a change.

After embarking on his life-changing weight-loss journey involving cooking Paleo meals, Bob's extreme bloating, acid reflux, dermatitis, and hematochezia (a condition that causes lower gastrointestinal bleeding) quickly subsided. "Within just three weeks of following a Paleo diet, my fears of needing surgery for my hematochezia were gone. The inflammation in my body decreased significantly," says Bob.

Today, Bob weighs in at a healthy 180 pounds. Following a Paleo diet has been the key to maintaining his weight loss and is an important part of his lifestyle since it inspired him to participate in a successful new business venture. He currently owns and operates the Not So Fast! Food Truck in San Diego, the first Paleo- and Primal-friendly food truck in California.

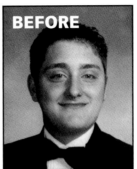

BEFORE

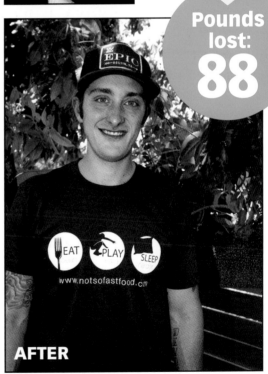

AFTER

Age: **31**

Height: **6'**

Weight before:
268

Weight after:
180

Pounds lost:
88

total cholesterol and bad LDL cholesterol—two measures of risk that were once believed to be the primary cause of heart disease. Investigators now know that other factors play as big a part in heart disease—things like inflammation, high levels of triglycerides (another type of blood fat), and low levels of good HDL cholesterol.

When saturated fat-containing foods are swapped for refined carbohydrates, inflammation worsens, triglycerides soar, and HDL cholesterol declines. Krauss concluded that there was no way to implicate saturated fat as the cause of heart disease.

Krauss's findings were part of the reason for the Copenhagen symposium on saturated fat. So were the results from the group at the Harvard School of Public Health. The experts reviewed the best evidence available—randomized clinical trials—and reported that saturated fat had a mixed, and mostly insignificant, effect on heart disease risk. Again, replacing saturated fat foods in the diet with those featuring carbohydrates or even monounsaturated fats offered no benefit.

A clear winner in this new world of dietary heroes and villains are polyunsaturated fatty acids—the fats that had a measurable benefit for the heart in the review of research. Paleo offers good sources of these fats, such as fish, nuts, and seeds. The researchers also believe that fiber-rich carbohydrates such as most fruits and vegetables are excellent choices.

The message, says Ronald Krauss, is to focus more on eating good food in reasonable amounts and less on how much fat—or what type—is in the food. "The only time I use the term low-fat is when I'm telling people to stop using the term."

So fat—especially saturated fat—has been given a reprieve. That's especially reassuring for the Paleo enthusiasts because the fats found in tropical foods such as coconuts and macadamia nuts tend to be saturated fat. (Of course, believing that plant foods that humans have eaten for thousands of years could somehow be harmful always seemed like a stretch.)

But what about the emphasis on protein that does exist in the Paleo plan? Is that really effective as a weight-loss strategy?

The answer is a resounding *yes*. In 2009, researchers at the University of Illinois and Penn State University conducted a 12-month university study of 130 people looking to shed some pounds. Half of them followed a high-carb, low-fat, low-protein diet inspired by the USDA food pyramid. The rest followed a diet moderately high in protein, about what you'll get on the 10 Pounds Off Paleo Diet.

The researchers taught the volunteers to shop and prepare meals based on the plan they were following, and then they tracked the dieters through an active four-month weight-loss phase and later for an additional eight months while the dieters attempted to maintain their loss.

After a year, the high-protein group had lost 23 percent more weight—and kept it off—than the low-fat dieters. It was a clear win for high-protein eating, but the news was even better than at first blush. When the researchers analyzed the volunteers' bodies, they discovered that the high-protein group had lost 22 percent more body fat during the four-month weight-loss phase compared to the low-fat group.

Even more remarkable, the high-protein group continued to shed body fat through the eight-month maintenance phase. At the end of 12 months, the high-protein dieters had lost 38 percent more body fat than the low-fat group. How could this happen? The researchers believe that the boost in filling, slow-to-digest protein helped control hunger and reduce snacking. The additional protein encouraged the growth of muscle; because muscles burn more calories than fat, the diet created a self-sustaining weight maintenance process, the researchers theorize.

The findings underline the true value of a higher-protein approach to weight loss: Yes, you'll lose more weight because you'll feel fuller than you would on a low-fat plan. But you'll also shed unhealthy and unsightly body fat while preserving your calorie-burning muscles. By the way, the other finding from the study was that, at year's end, more than half of the low-fat group had dropped out of the study, while two-thirds of the high-protein dieters were still going strong. The bottom line: Paleo is the quickest, most effective, and easiest way to get the vibrant body you want.

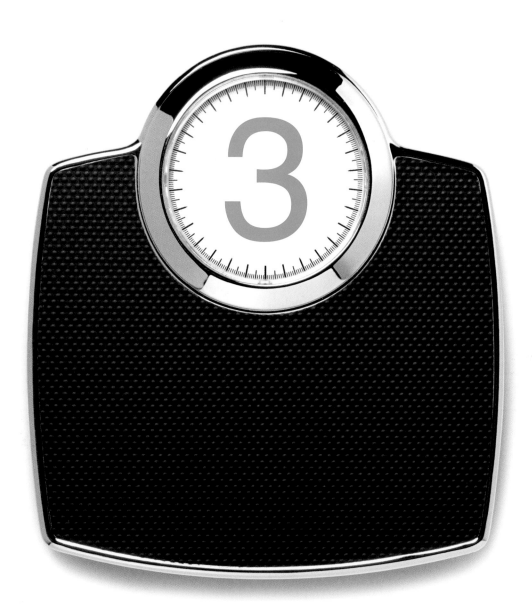

THE NUTS AND BOLTS OF GOING PALEO

ONE WAY TO THINK OF THE PALEO plan is to imagine yourself on a deserted tropical island: Anything you can catch and kill, pick, or forage is good. Wild animals? Yes. Fish? Eat away. Pineapple, coconut, and any other fruit you can find—dive in. Seeds and nuts are also on the menu, as are eggs.

But dairy, cereal grains, refined sugar and fats, fast food, and processed foods like frozen dinners are all off limits since there's no way you could procure these items on your island. If that seems too restrictive, breathe easy. You'll quickly adjust to this new way of eating, and you'll feel so good you'll wonder why you ever ate junk.

Meat

You may wonder why Paleo emphasizes wild game and grass-fed, free-range meat. Grass-fed livestock contains a better mix of fats.

Farmers have found that if they let cows or sheep graze a field of mixed grass and grains, the animals will carefully eat around the grain to get at the grass. It's their natural food, yet today most feed animals are raised on grain. Why? For the same reason you're trying to avoid grain: It helps fatten the animals up more quickly. All that grain feed also alters the mix of fats in the meat, depressing levels of heart-healthy omega-3 fatty acids. Feeding animals grains also increases the overall fat content of the animals.

A recent study revealed that meat cuts from grass-fed animals contain almost 60 percent less fat than cuts from grain-fed livestock. While it's getting easier to find free-range, grass-fed meat these days, you may have to pay a bit more.

FOOD SWAP

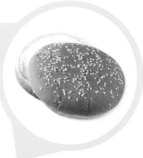

✘ Replace hamburger buns
✔ with portobello mushrooms.

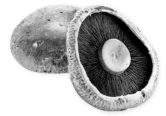

BETTER BUNS Believe it or not, those generous portobello mushroom caps can step in perfectly for hamburger buns and other sandwich breads. Remove the stem, scrape out the gills from under the cap, and set them aside. (You can use these to top a salad or mix them in with the burger meat.) Fry them in olive oil for a few minutes to crisp them up, and then set them aside to cool while you prepare the burger. You'll find the caps will hold your toppings on your burger much better than a traditional bun, plus they increase the overall nutrition value in your meal.

Basically, any wild game makes the Paleo meat list. These animals have a preferential mix of fats, and their meat tends to be much leaner than feedlot-raised animals. Seafood makes the list because it's especially high in healthy fats, and it tends to be naturally lean. Eggs may not be a meat, but they make the list since they're nearly a perfect protein. They're loaded with healthy fats and important nutrients, and they're inexpensive.

Beef	Lamb	Turkey
Bison	Mutton	Venison
Chicken	Pork	Wild-caught fish
Eggs	Shellfish	

Paleo Vegetables and Fruits

These need little explanation: Almost any sensible diet promotes regular consumption of produce. There are some limits when it comes to Paleo, though, but you'll hear about those later.

VEGETABLES

Artichokes	Dandelion greens	Pumpkins
Asparagus	Eggplant	Radishes
Beet Greens	Endive	Seaweed
Beets	Green onions	Spinach
Bell Peppers	Kale	Squash
Broccoli	Kohlrabi	Swiss chard
Brussels sprouts	Lettuce	Tomatillos
Cabbage	Mushrooms	Tomatoes
Carrots	Mustard Greens	Turnips
Cauliflower	Onions	Yams/sweet potatoes
Celery	Parsley	Watercress
Collard greens	Parsnips	
Cucumbers	Peppers (spicy)	

FRUITS

Apples	Guavas	Papayas
Apricots	Kiwis	Passion fruit
Avocados	Lemons	Peaches
Bananas	Limes	Pears
Berries (all types)	Lychees	Pineapples
Cherries	Mangoes	Plums
Figs	Melons (all types)	Pomegranates
Grapefruit	Nectarines	Star fruit
Grapes	Oranges	Tangerines

PALEO NUTS AND SEEDS

These are nature's protein-and-nutrient powerhouses. They'll give salads some heft, ground up they serve as flour or butter, or you can just snack on them.

Almonds	Macadamia nuts	Pumpkinseeds
Brazil nuts	Pecans	Sesame seeds
Cashews	Pine nuts	Sunflower seeds
Hazelnuts	Pistachios	Walnuts

PALEO OILS

The story on cooking oils is a bit complicated. All the oils you've been told are healthy—canola, sunflower, safflower—are actually unusually high in omega-6 fatty acids. There's nothing wrong with these fats as long as they're in balance with omega-3 fatty acids. The problem with many vegetable oils is that they have primarily omega-6s. To help get your diet back into balance, look for oils that have a healthy balance or favor omega-3 fatty acids.

Avocado	Ghee (clarified butter)
Butter from grass-fed cows	Nut oils/butters
Coconut	Olive

Foods to Avoid

These are relatively easy to remember. Basically, the entire dairy category is eliminated on Paleo, though some people like to keep some cheeses—goat or hard cheeses like Parmesan—around. These are fermented long enough to remove the lactose sugars that can cause digestive troubles for some people. Kefir and yogurt are also on the "maybe" list, but otherwise you'll want to avoid milk-based products.

Be doubly sure to check ingredient labels for products that might be made with dairy.

CEREAL GRAINS are also off the list for the reasons listed in the previous chapter. The things to watch for on labels include:

Amaranth	Millet	Rye
Barley	Oats	Sorghum
Buckwheat	Quinoa	Wheat
Corn	Rice	Wild rice

LEGUMES are also no-nos, mostly because they're loaded with starches and enzymes that can cause inflammation and difficulty digesting. (There's a reason they're known as the magical fruit.) Just remember that peanuts are a legume, not a nut, so they make the list, as do peas, soybeans, and all the things made with soy (such as tofu). For many of the same reasons, starchy vegetables such as potatoes, cassava root, manioc, and tapioca are also off the list. (Yams get the OK, because they contain plenty of valuable nutrients that justify their presence in your diet.)

Along with all the processed food and drinks that you'll be avoiding in the future, make sure to avoid diet soda and artificial sweeteners. While these might seem harmless, they're far from it. You might think you can save calories by eating foods or drinking sodas flavored with artificial sweeteners. But the savings are illusory.

When Harvard researchers tracked people who primarily drank artificially sweetened beverages, they discovered that the diet soda drinkers gained more weight than people who drank regular soda (though both groups put on pounds).

Back in the lab, the researchers discovered that when rats are given artificial sweeteners they actually eat more food than rats that get real sugar, possibly because calorie sensors in the gut and brain expect to gain energy from such a sweet taste. When the calories fail to turn up, these sensors prompted the rats to overeat to compensate. The saccharin taste of these artificial sweeteners—which are as much as a hundred times sweeter than the taste of sugar—presents another problem, say experts. We're training our taste buds to expect extreme flavors, and simple good sweet food like fruit pales in comparison. We end up shunning it in favor of the sensationally sweet foods. Cut out the diet soda—and the regular soda.

You'll miss them initially, but you can replace the drinks with seltzer sweetened with a splash of fruit juice or flavored with a squeeze of lemon or lime. Within a week or two your taste buds will have recalibrated themselves, and you'll get more pleasure from a truly healthy and weight-loss-friendly diet.

Smart Food Tips

FLOUR POWER Refined white flour is out for baking, but you'll find that almond flour can fill in nicely when you're making muffins or other baked goods. It's gluten free and much higher in nutrients than wheat flour.

SUGAR SUBSTITUTE No, not Splenda. Instead of using refined white sugar in your recipes, coffee, or baked goods, try raw honey or pure maple syrup instead. They're plenty sweet, they're natural, and they'll add flavor beyond simple sweetness.

PEANUT BUTTER Despite the name, peanuts are not nuts. But almonds are, and so are sunflowers. You can find actual nut and seed butters relatively easily these days, and using them as spreads or in smoothies is a great way to get filling, Paleo-friendly fats and proteins into your morning repast.

BABA GHANOUSH Although eggplant, the primary ingredient in this dip, is Paleo-friendly, store-bought concoctions may contain no-nos like mayonnaise. Make your own by grilling or roasting the eggplants until the skin darkens. Cool, peel, and then blend with garlic, olive oil, cumin, and salt and pepper. For more authentic flavor, add some tahini, which is ground sesame seed paste.

SALAD DRESSING STAND-INS
Oil and vinegar are the perfect Paleo dressing, but beware of pre-packaged versions, which contain tons of sugar and preservatives and may not be made with olive oil. Whip up your own instead, and mix in some pressed garlic, sea salt, and pepper to taste. If you're missing Ranch dressing, try a version with soaked raw cashews and coconut milk: Pulse ¹/₂ cup of the cashews in a food processor until you get a paste, and then mix in a cup of coconut milk, some garlic and onion powder, lemon juice, sea salt, pepper, and dried dillweed.

HARD CIDER IS EASY When you're craving a libation, consider hard cider. Perhaps the most Paleo-friendly form of alcohol, it's fermented—excellent—

FOOD SWAP

✘ Replace fries
✔ with carrot fries.

CRAVING FRIES? Try carrot fries instead. Slice up some carrots into sticks, toss with olive oil and sea salt, and then bake them at 425 degrees until they're crisp. Sprinkle on some herbs of your choice, and you'll find they rival potato fries for flavor.

and usually made from apples. You'll have to check labels to make sure it's gluten free, and choose dry cider to cut down on the added sugar.

HAVE YOUR CAKE Thanks to hard work by Paleo enthusiasts, you can find recipes for occasional sweet indulgences like cakes, cookies, and even banana bread without too much trouble, including several right here in this book, beginning on page 166. Almond flour, coconut oil, and maple syrup will be the trick to producing baked goods anyone—Paleo or not—can love.

COZY UP TO CACAO This is the beanlike seed that is the origin of the chocolate you love so dearly. The raw, organic versions are cold-pressed and loaded with healthy nutrients and enzymes that studies have linked to a lower risk of heart disease and diabetes. Spend some time figuring out how much maple syrup or honey it takes to produce a rich chocolate flavor; this is experimentation anyone can appreciate.

> "Not only did I lose 70 pounds after following the Paleo lifestyle, but my life was changed forever."

Success Story:
Chae

At age 22 and with the scale topping at over 300 pounds, Chae began her own physical transformation from an unhealthy woman with a life full of bad habits to one who is happy and strong! While in college and studying abroad in Australia, she adopted a healthier lifestyle by cooking nutritious foods at home and walking regularly. When she returned stateside one year later, she weighed 70 pounds lighter, gained a new perspective, and began to feel self-love. Later she began eating a diet focused on whole foods and dropped another 70 pounds.

Her new way of life allowed her to reverse the symptoms of psoriasis, eczema, and alopecia areata. Today, 140 pounds lighter, she is strong, happy, and spreading awareness about her healthy lifestyle. "I fully believe that the way we feed ourselves is reflected in not just our physical and mental health, but in the health of our spirit, the health of our relationships with others, and the health of our connection to the Earth."

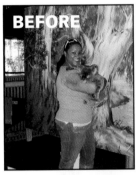

BEFORE

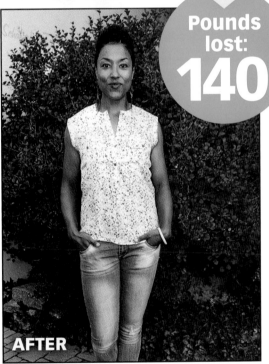

AFTER

Age: **30**

Height: **5'9"**

Weight before:
300

Weight after:
160

Pounds lost:
140

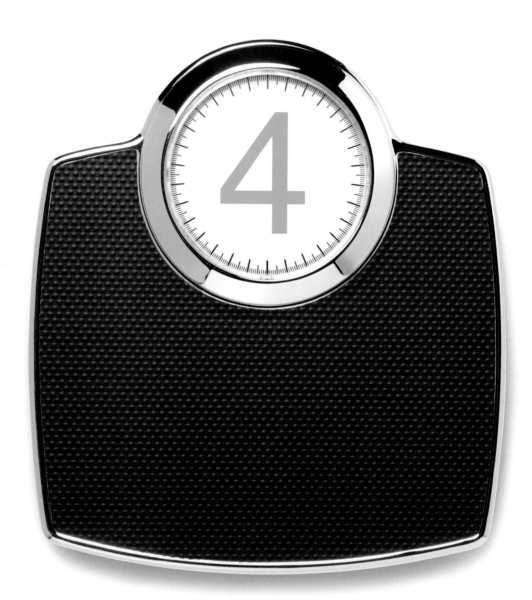

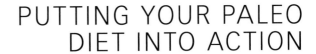

PUTTING YOUR PALEO DIET INTO ACTION

NOW THAT YOU KNOW what you can and can't eat on your Paleo diet, it's time to clear out your kitchen. Contact a local shelter or food pantry to see if they'll accept donations, and then collect some boxes and garbage bags. Now you're ready to purge.

Go for the cereal boxes, the bags of white flour and sugar, the sodas, the peanut butter, and the gallons of milk. Look for the cans of soup, stew, and chili, and don't forget the jarred pasta sauces and packaged noodle mixes. Clear out the bagels and bread, the cookies and ice cream, and the packages of pasta. Anything with an ingredient list of more than five items is suspect. If sugar, wheat, corn, milk, or any of the other off-limits foods is one of those ingredients, the food must go. If the food is unopened, you might be able to donate it; a neighbor or relative might be open to taking the rest.

Paleo Spices

Once you've cleared the shelves, take a look at Chapter 6 (beginning on page 60) for a shopping list of Paleo-friendly basics that you'll want to stock your cabinets with. One area you'll want to be sure is well stocked: your spice rack. Now that you'll be preparing more of your meals from scratch, spices are your ally. Alphabetize your spices since you'll be reaching for them much more often. Here's a primer list:

Bay leaves	Garlic powder
Cardamom	Ginger
Cayenne pepper	Ground mustard
Chives	Mint
Cinnamon	Oregano
Cloves	Paprika
Cocoa	Pepper
Coriander	Salt
Cumin	Thyme

You may want to consider planting an herb garden as well. You can even grow herbs indoors with new kits on the market, and there's nothing like fresh basil, cilantro, rosemary, and thyme to liven up a dish.

Paleo Tools

You probably have plenty of kitchen appliances on hand, but peruse this list to see if you're missing anything. While these items aren't essential, they will make preparing meals for your new eating plan much simpler.

8-INCH CAST-IRON SKILLET You'll find this skillet is perfect for whipping up some uncured ham and eggs for breakfast. These pans typically come preseasoned, so all you have to do is be sure to keep it in shape. Use coconut oils, ghee, or organic butter when you cook; rinse the skillet—no soap!—right after you finish, and use a dishwashing brush to knock off the food scraps. Thoroughly dry the pan, and smear a little of your cooking oil all over the top and bottom. Keep the skillet in a dry place that's handy. Food simply tastes better when made in these pans, and the care is so simple that you'll wonder why you ever bothered with so-called no-stick cookware (and all the chemicals!).

EGG POACHERS One thing you'll be eating a lot more of when you start Paleo is eggs. You may tire of fried, scrambled, and hard-boiled, which is why having egg poachers on hand will keep your breakfasts feeling fresh. You can get silicone cups that float in boiling water, allowing you to cook poached eggs to perfection. Mix poached eggs with some quick-braised greens for a healthy, Paleo-friendly start to your day.

IMMERSION BLENDER This will come in handy morning, noon, and night. You can use it to mix up a personal smoothie in the morning to set you up for the day. Or you can use it to mix sauces and salad dressings.

10- OR 12-INCH CAST-IRON SKILLET Again, this will be your go-to pan for cooking most of your dinner meals, whether it's searing steaks, crisping roasts that you'll finish in the oven (the great advantage of these pans is they can easily go from the stove top to the oven and back again), or whipping up stir-fries. Unlike most cookware, these hardy pans improve with age, and their seasoning adds flavor to everything you cook.

When you've transferred your meal to a serving dish, run the pan under hot water while you give it a quick scrub with a long-handled stiff-bristled plastic brush. Dry, smear with a little coconut oil or ghee, and put it away until the next time you need it.

BAKING SHEETS Roasting vegetables like cauliflower, asparagus, and broccoli with olive oil, garlic, and pepper turns them into gourmet delights. Kale chips are a great stand-in for potato chips. But to pull these dishes off with ease and panache, you'll need a good supply of baking sheets. Keep your cleanup quick and easy by lining the sheets with foil or parchment paper before baking.

QUALITY KNIVES A sharp knife is a blessing in the kitchen. It turns a prep job from a chore to a pleasure, and the sharper the better: A dull knife is far more likely to slip and slice your finger than a sharp one. (So consider a quality sharpener to help maintain the edges.) You can spend hundreds of dollars per knife, but *America's Test Kitchen* found that the relatively inexpensive Victorinox Fibrox kitchen knives fared just as well as far more expensive German brands.

SPIRALIZER This device can do wonderful things with vegetables to help them fill in for the grain foods you may be missing. You can turn squash, carrots, and other firm veggies into noodles for a pasta substitute, noodles in a soup, or an interesting textured filling in a lettuce wrap.

DIGITAL THERMOMETER When you'll be preparing lots of meat, this is an invaluable tool. The digital versions can give you a much faster read; some include the option of leaving the sensor in the meat in the oven and the readout on the counter.

STOCKPOT If you aren't making your own stock, now's the time to start. The store-bought stuff is unreasonably salty and usually loaded with chemicals. Drop a leftover chicken carcass or beef bones, roughly chopped onions, celery, carrots, and your choice of spices into a stockpot full of water, and let it simmer for an hour or so—you'll have the best stock you've ever had. Choose a big pot—20 quarts isn't too big. (You can always freeze your leftover stock.)

FOOD PROCESSOR When you need to puree a lot of soup or prepare a large quantity of sauce, these are hard to beat. You can also grind meat and slice or grate vegetables with one of these.

SLOW COOKER The simplest way to save yourself time at the end of the day is to make dinner in the morning. Throw a bunch of fresh ingredients into your cooker along with broth and some bay leaves before you leave for work. Voilà: At the end of the day your dinner is ready, and your house will smell wonderful.

GOOD STORAGE CONTAINERS Prepare double or triple batches of your favorite meals, and freeze the leftovers in high-quality, freezer-durable containers. That's one or more meals you won't have to prepare down the road!

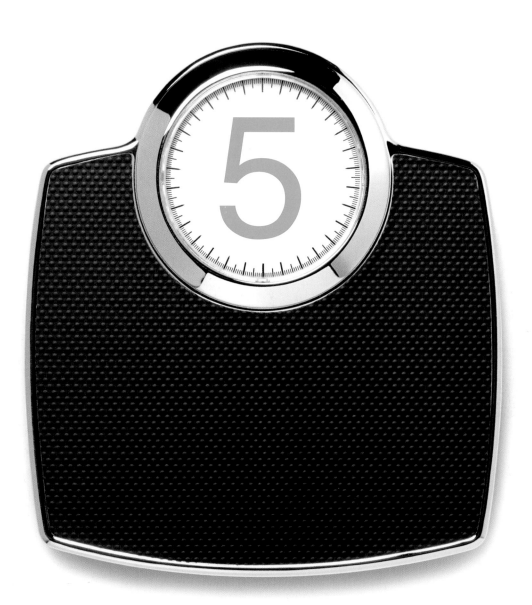

EADY TO DIVE IN? Your kitchen is prepared, you have the food you need, and now it's time to take the challenge. In this chapter, you'll find four weeks of food plans that will help you lose at least the 10 pounds you want to drop. You may find that you'll drop even more. You'll also feel better, especially if you add the exercise component from Chapter 12. All the meals are referenced by page number. If you find dishes that really work for your taste buds and your time budget, feel free to stick with those.

WEEK 1

	BREAKFAST	LUNCH	DINNER
MONDAY	Sunshine Smoothie (pg. 83)	Chicken Lettuce Cups (pg. 87)	Baked Citrus-Herb Salmon (pg. 110)
TUESDAY	Watermelon-Blueberry Salad (pg. 81)	Beefy Jicama Wraps (pg. 90)	Spicy-Sweet Chicken Thighs with Roasted Asparagus (pg. 125)
WEDNESDAY	Cantaloupe with Honey and Lime (pg. 76)	Tuna, Artichoke, and Roasted Red Pepper Wrap (pg. 92)	Beef Fillets with Rosemary Sauce (pg. 131)
THURSDAY	Raspberry-Banana Smoothie (pg. 82)	Seared Steak Salad (pg. 103)	Scallops with Tomato-Herb Broth (pg. 114)
FRIDAY	Baked Eggs with Kale Sauté (pg. 70)	Cajun Chicken Stew (pg. 93)	Beef Chili (pg. 127)
SATURDAY	Mushroom Frittata (pg. 73)	Shrimp and Herb Salad (pg. 101)	Citrus-Herb Chicken (pg. 115)
SUNDAY	Gingered Tropical Fruit Salad (pg. 178)	Easy Vegetable-Beef Soup (pg. 95)	Spicy Shrimp and Avocado Salad with Mango Vinaigrette (pg. 113)

WEEK 2

	BREAKFAST	LUNCH	DINNER
MONDAY	**Raspberry-Banana Smoothie** (pg. 82)	**Lamb Picadillo Wrap** (pg. 91)	**Maple-Mustard Glazed Chicken** (pg. 119)
TUESDAY	**Blueberry Citrus Salad** (pg. 80)	**Chicken and Mint Coleslaw Wraps** (pg. 88)	**Pan-Seared Snapper with Garlic-Herb Vinaigrette** (pg. 111)
WEDNESDAY	**Baked Eggs with Chopped Tomato and Chives** (pg. 69)	**Chicken and Lettuce Salad with Orange Dressing** (pg. 98)	**Spiced Pork Chops with Butternut Squash** (pg. 138)
THURSDAY	**Berry-Ginger Salad** (pg. 79)	**Cajun Chicken Stew** (pg. 93)	**Steak Florentine** (pg. 129)
FRIDAY	**Honey-Glazed Plums with Almonds** (pg. 77)	**Beefy Jicama Wraps** (pg. 90)	**Spicy Herb-Rubbed Grilled Chicken** (pg. 120)
SATURDAY	**Summer Vegetable Frittata** (pg. 74)	**Thai Seafood Salad** (pg. 99)	**Rosemary Lamb Chops with Garlic-Balsamic Sauce** (pg. 141)
SUNDAY	**Baked Eggs with Canadian Bacon** (pg. 71)	**Asian Tenderloin Salad** (pg. 102)	**Steak and Avocado Kebabs** (pg. 133)

WEEK 3

	BREAKFAST	LUNCH	DINNER
MONDAY	Sunshine Smoothie (pg. 83)	Guacamole Chicken Wraps (pg. 89)	Grilled Cumin Chicken with Tomatillo Sauce (pg. 122)
TUESDAY	Berry-Ginger Salad (pg. 79)	Beefy Jicama Wraps (pg. 90)	Cilantro-Lime Chicken with Avocado Salsa (pg. 121)
WEDNESDAY	Baked Eggs with Kale Sauté (pg. 70)	Coconut Shrimp Soup (pg. 97)	Beef with Carrots and Dried Plums (pg. 128)
THURSDAY	Raspberry-Banana Smoothie (pg. 82)	Chicken Lettuce Cups (pg. 87)	Halibut à la Provençal over Mixed Greens (pg. 109)
FRIDAY	Watermelon-Blueberry Salad (pg. 81)	Easy Vegetable-Beef Soup (pg. 95)	Chicken Kebabs and Nectarine Salsa (pg. 117)
SATURDAY	Turkey Breakfast Sausage (pg. 71)	Chicken and Lettuce Salad with Orange Dressing (pg. 98)	Beef Tenderloin with Chimichurri Sauce (pg. 134)
SUNDAY	Baked Frittata Ribbons in Tomato Sauce (pg. 68)	Gazpacho with Lemon-Garlic Shrimp (pg. 96)	Slider Patties with Pomegranate Molasses (pg. 140)

	BREAKFAST	LUNCH	DINNER
MONDAY	Raspberry-Banana Smoothie (pg. 82)	Cajun Chicken Stew (pg. 93)	Arctic Char with Orange-Caper Relish (pg. 107)
TUESDAY	Baked Eggs with Chopped Tomato and Chives (pg. 69)	Tuna, Artichoke, and Roasted Red Pepper Wrap (pg. 92)	Pork Medallions with Herbed Mushroom Sauce (pg. 135)
WEDNESDAY	Blueberry Citrus Salad (pg. 80)	Lamb Picadillo Wrap (pg. 91)	Italian-Seasoned Roast Chicken Breasts (pg. 116)
THURSDAY	Prosciutto-Wrapped Melon Slices (pg. 75)	Coconut Shrimp Soup (pg. 97)	Chicken Thighs with Cilantro-Mint Chutney (pg. 123)
FRIDAY	Honey-Glazed Plums with Almonds (pg. 77)	Asian Tenderloin Salad (pg. 102)	Chicken Kebabs and Nectarine Salsa (pg. 117)
SATURDAY	Summer Vegetable Frittata (pg. 74)	Thai Seafood Salad (pg. 99)	Lemon-Herb Skillet Pork Chops (pg. 139)
SUNDAY	Poached Eggs with Spinach and Walnuts (pg. 67)	Shrimp and Herb Salad (pg. 101)	New York Strip with Carrots (pg. 132)

Snacks

There are a couple of recipes for snacks (check out Deviled Eggs, page 145; Kale Chips, page 146; and Masala Pumpkinseeds, page 149), but for the most part, you'll want to experiment to find the snacks that work best in terms of filling you up and satisfying your cravings. Here are some other ideas you can experiment with:

Fresh fruit	Dried fruit
Homemade beef jerky	Hard-boiled eggs
Raw vegetables	Nuts or seeds
Guacamole	Slices of beef, chicken, or turkey

Dessert

Pleasing your sweet tooth is easier than you might think on a Paleo plan—just be sure not to overindulge so that you can reach your weight loss goals. You'll find plenty of dessert options in Chapter 11 (page 164). When you don't have time to prepare a special dessert, dark chocolate is almost completely Paleo compliant—stick to a square at a time to satisfy your craving for sweets.

Eating Out with Paleo

It's all too easy to have trouble staying true to your Paleo plan when eating out. These tips can help you navigate most menus and restaurants with ease.

- **Get to know your server/chef.** If you're eating out near your place of work, you probably have two or three places you go to regularly. Don't hesitate to ask questions about how the food is prepared to make sure it conforms to your new diet.
- **Ask about gluten-free options.** Most restaurants are ready to accommodate people who are gluten intolerant, and these dishes will usually fit nicely into your Paleo plan.

- **Order the burger minus the bun**. Most restaurants will be happy to prepare your meal minus the bread if you ask nicely.
- **Ask the server to not bring the bread**. You'll find it a lot easier to avoid bread if it never comes to the table. You'll have to get your dining companions to agree, but most people are happy to avoid the extra needless calories from pre-meal bread or tortilla chips.
- **Ask that the food be cooked in olive oil**. Although you'll have a tough time finding mainstream restaurants that cook with ghee or coconut oil, almost every industrial kitchen will have plenty of olive oil on hand. Ask if your dish can be prepared using the healthier choice.
- **Get veggies for your sides**. Almost every entrée seems to come with potatoes or French fries. But any decent restaurant will be happy to substitute some steamed or olive oil-fried veggies.
- **Beware of added sugar**. Chefs know that an easy way to liven up a sauce is to add sugar. If you're ordering something that comes with a sauce, ask about the sugar—and the flour—content before saying yes.
- **Don't stress too much**. At the end of the day you want to enjoy your evening out. Remember that your meal is more about enjoying the atmosphere and your companions than it is about adhering to your plan. If you slip up at this one meal, don't sweat it too much. You can get back on your plan when you're back in control of the preparation.

Eating on the Run Paleo-Style

While preparing a beautiful meal and cooking more at home is what Paleo is all about, the pressures of modern life often get in the way. Here are some ideas for quick breakfasts and lunches.

- **Hard-Boiled Eggs** This is the ultimate simple on-the-go Paleo breakfast. Mix it with some fresh fruit or kale chips, and you can start your day with a solid blast of nutrients and protein.
- **Smoothie** Throw some kale or spinach or lower-sugar fruits like frozen

berries, pineapple, or mango; and ice into a blender for a smoothie that you can drink on your way to work and will get you through your morning.

• **Breakfast Bars** You might be able to find Paleo-friendly breakfast bars at your local grocer, but you will be better off making your own (so you can control the sugar and calories). Some examples include cinnamon breakfast bars or banana ginger bars made with coconut flour and honey or maple syrup.

• **Breakfast Burritos** Keep some cooked sausage alongside your hard-boiled eggs for those days when you're in a rush. Crumble the eggs and slice the sausage over a cabbage leaf or a coconut flour tortilla. (For the tortilla, blend three egg whites with half a tablespoon of coconut flour and your favorite seasonings, such as garlic power or cilantro for savory, or cinnamon and a teaspoon or 2 of honey for a sweet role. Pour the mixture into a hot greased skillet, and cover. Cook until set; then flip and cook for a few seconds more.)

• **Paleo Cereal** Bring along a baggie of this mixture to nosh on: chopped almonds, chia seeds, coconut flakes, and some dried mango. If you have time to actually sit down to a bowl of cereal, you can pour $1/4$ cup coconut milk over about $1/2$ cup nut and fruit mixture.

• **Bell Pepper Sandwiches** Slice bell pepper into wide, flat slabs, and make sandwiches with sliced turkey, pitted olives, and greens of your choice.

• **Last Night's Leftovers** That delicious steak can be sliced up and rolled into a cabbage burrito for the following day's lunch.

• **Veggies and Dip** Bring pieces of carrot, celery, broccoli, and cauliflower to dip in a tablespoon or 2 of almond butter or guacamole.

Traveling with Paleo

When you're on the road, you'll face a lot of temptations to leave your Paleo diet behind. If you give in from time to time, don't sweat it; you can get back on track when you get home, and the last thing you want to do is add stress to a vacation or business trip. One easy way to cover yourself is to pack a lot of snacks—they'll get you through situations where finding a Paleo option may be tough. Here are some other tricks to keep in mind.

- **Find a diner first**. If you can get a good Paleo breakfast to start your day, your battle is well on the way to being won. For that reason, a diner is your friend. They'll always have a meat and eggs option, and you should be able to get some fruit on the side and orange or grapefruit juice.

- **Know your cuisines.** Mexican food can be very Paleo friendly if you resist the beans, tortillas, and chips. Fajitas are a Paleo slam dunk. Sushi restaurants will allow you to order the sashimi—no rice—and you can even substitute the soy sauce for tamari sauce, which is gluten free. Steakhouses are always a good option. Just avoid Italian and country-style French places.

- **Aim for 70-80 percent Paleo.** Let's face it, when you're traveling, it will be tough to maintain your Paleo guidelines. Try as much as possible to hit the target, but don't worry about the 20-30 percent of the time when it's just not possible to be strictly Paleo.

PART 2

100 PALEO RECIPES

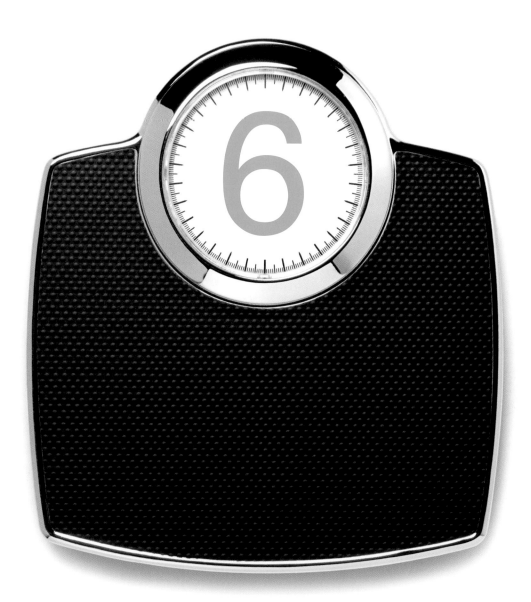

PALEO SHOPPING LIST

KEEPING YOUR PANTRY WELL STOCKED with Paleo-friendly food will make following this plan much easier. You'll be able to cook up any number of tasty meals at a moment's notice with the right food and seasonings on hand. Making your own meals from scratch is a big part of Paleo, so you can't neglect your kitchen.

In the previous chapters, we talked about some handy kitchen utensils that make producing Paleo meals a breeze. That's the same with these foods: They allow you to whip up great meals without effort. Some of these foods you'll need to eat and replace weekly; others keep for months. The more you experiment with the recipes, meals, and snacks that work for you, the better sense you'll have of what you need to shop for.

Paleo Pantry and Shopping List

MEAT (REFRIGERATOR OR FREEZER)

__ Beef	__ Bison	__ Chicken
__ Deli meat (nitrite free, sugar free)	__ Duck	__ Eggs
	__ Fish, Shellfish	__ Lamb
__ Organ meats	__ Pork	__ Quail
__ Sausage (nitrite free, sugar free)	__ Turkey	__ Veal
	__ Venison	

VEGETABLES

__ Artichoke	__ Arugula	__ Asparagus
__ Beets, Beet greens	__ Bell peppers	__ Bok choy
__ Broccoli	__ Brussels sprouts	__ Cabbage
__ Carrots	__ Cauliflower	__ Celery
__ Chile peppers	__ Collard greens	__ Cucumber
__ Eggplant	__ Endive	__ Escarole
__ Garlic	__ Green beans	__ Kale
__ Kohlrabi	__ Leeks	__ Lettuce
__ Mushrooms	__ Mustard greens	__ Nori (seaweed)
__ Okra	__ Onion	__ Parsnip
__ Pumpkin	__ Radish	__ Shallots
__ Snow peas	__ Spinach	__ Squash (all varieties)
__ Sweet potatoes	__ Tomatoes	__ Tomatillos
__ Turnips	__ Yams	

FRUITS

- __ Apples
- __ Apricots
- __ Bananas
- __ Blackberries
- __ Blueberries
- __ Cantaloupe
- __ Cherries
- __ Clementines
- __ Cranberries
- __ Dates
- __ Figs
- __ Grapefruit
- __ Grapes
- __ Honeydew
- __ Kiwi
- __ Kumquats
- __ Lemons
- __ Limes
- __ Lychees
- __ Mandarin oranges
- __ Mangoes
- __ Nectarines
- __ Oranges
- __ Papayas
- __ Peaches
- __ Pears
- __ Pineapple
- __ Plums
- __ Pomegranates
- __ Raspberries
- __ Tangerines
- __ Watermelon

FATS AND OILS

- __ Almond butter
- __ Cashew butter
- __ Clarified butter
- __ Coconut butter
- __ Coconut oil
- __ Ghee
- __ Hazelnut butter
- __ Olive oil
- __ Palm shortening

SEASONINGS, FLAVORINGS, AND BAKING SUPPLIES

- __ Almond meal
- __ Avocado oil
- __ Broth/stock
- __ Chiles, dried (variety)
- __ Coconut aminos
- __ Coconut, shredded and unsweetened
- __ Coconut flour
- __ Curry paste
- __ Gingerroot (frozen)
- __ Fish sauce
- __ Herbs, fresh and dried
- __ Honey
- __ Maple syrup
- __ Peppercorns
- __ Sea salt
- __ Spices
- __ Tomatoes, canned (paste, chopped, sauce)

SNACKS

- __ Almonds
- __ Apricots, dried
- __ Brazil nuts
- __ Cashews
- __ Cranberries, dried
- __ Hazelnuts
- __ Jerky
- __ Macadamia nuts
- __ Pecans
- __ Pistachios
- __ Plums, dried
- __ Raisins
- __ Walnuts

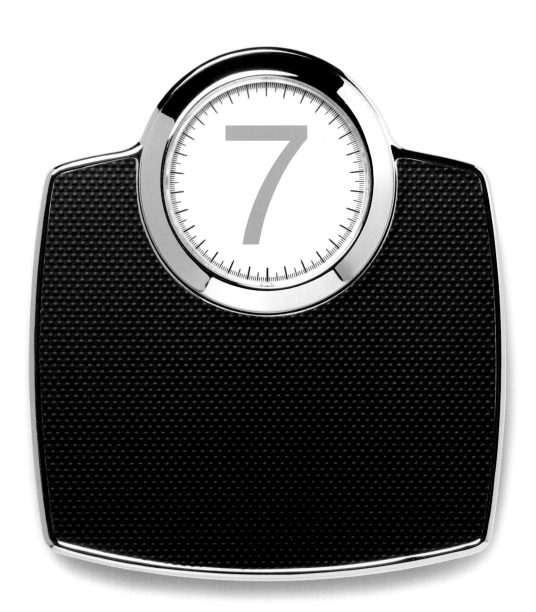

START YOUR DAY RIGHT BY

eating a filling breakfast! Whether you are pressed for time or can sit down to have a relaxing meal, you'll find plenty of options to give you the energy you need to jumpstart your day. From quick smoothies to fresh fruit medleys and hearty egg bakes to easy homemade chicken sausage, a delicious breakfast will always be within reach.

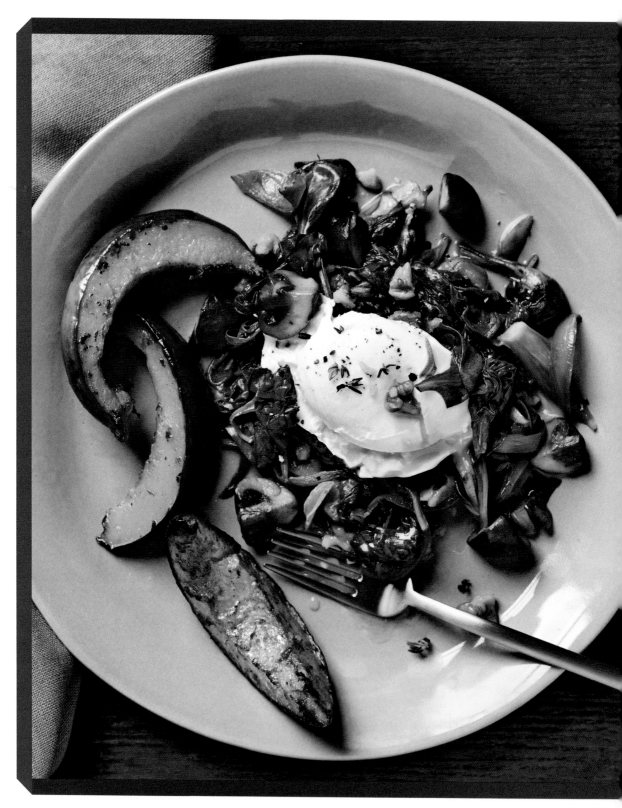

Poached Eggs with Spinach and Walnuts

Serve protein-packed eggs over a side of spinach sautéed with mushrooms and walnuts.

1	tablespoon olive oil, divided
1	(10-ounce) bag baby spinach, chopped
3	garlic cloves, minced
3	vertically sliced shallots
1	tablespoon chopped fresh sage
¾	teaspoon chopped thyme, divided
½	teaspoon black pepper, divided
¼	teaspoon salt
1	(8-ounce) package cremini mushrooms, quartered
¾	cup toasted walnuts, chopped and divided
2	tablespoons red wine vinegar
8	cups water
2	tablespoons white vinegar
4	large eggs

1. Heat a large Dutch oven over medium-high heat. Add 1 teaspoon oil. Add spinach; sauté 2 minutes. Remove spinach from pan; drain, cool slightly, and squeeze out excess moisture. Add remaining oil to pan. Add garlic and shallots; sauté 3 minutes. Add sage, ½ teaspoon thyme, ¼ teaspoon pepper, salt, and mushrooms; sauté 7 minutes. Stir in spinach, ½ cup walnuts, and red wine vinegar; cook 30 seconds.

2. Combine 8 cups water and white vinegar in a large saucepan, and bring to a simmer. Break each egg gently into pan. Cook 3 minutes. Remove eggs using a slotted spoon. Spoon ²/₃ cup mushroom mixture onto each of 4 plates. Top each serving with 1 egg. Sprinkle evenly with remaining thyme, pepper, and walnuts.

YIELD | SERVES 4

CALORIES 350; FAT 24.3g (sat 5.5g, mono 7.5g, poly 10.2g); PROTEIN 17g; CARB 18g; FIBER 5g; CHOL 196mg; IRON 4mg; SODIUM 383mg; CALC 257mg

Baked Frittata Ribbons in Tomato Sauce

Sauce:

Cooking spray

2   **cups finely chopped onion**

2   **tablespoons finely chopped fresh flat-leaf parsley**

2   **tablespoons finely chopped fresh basil**

2   **garlic cloves, minced**

4   **cups chopped, seeded, peeled plum tomatoes (about 2½ pounds)**

½   **teaspoon salt**

Frittata:

¼   **cup finely chopped fresh flat-leaf parsley**

½   **teaspoon salt**

¼   **teaspoon freshly ground black pepper**

4   **large eggs**

4   **large egg whites**

1. To prepare sauce, heat a large nonstick skillet over medium heat. Coat pan with cooking spray. Add onion, 2 tablespoons parsley, basil, and garlic; cook 7 minutes or until onion is tender, stirring frequently. Stir in the tomatoes and ½ teaspoon salt. Cover, reduce heat to medium-low, and cook 15 minutes, stirring occasionally. Preheat broiler.

2. To prepare frittata, combine ¼ cup parsley and remaining ingredients, stirring with a whisk until well blended. Heat a large nonstick skillet over medium-high heat; coat pan with cooking spray. Add half of egg mixture, and cook 2 minutes or until bottom is set. Carefully turn frittata over. Cook 1 minute.

3. Place cooked frittata on a cutting board. Repeat procedure with remaining egg mixture.

4. Roll up cooked frittatas, jelly-roll fashion, and cut into ¼-inch-thick slices. Combine sauce and frittata ribbons in a medium bowl, tossing to coat. Divide the frittata mixture evenly among 6 (6-ounce) ramekins or custard cups. Broil 2 minutes or until mixture is thoroughly heated.

YIELD | SERVES 6 (SERVING SIZE: 1 RAMEKIN)

CALORIES 126; FAT 5g (sat 1.8g, mono 1.7g, poly 0.7g); PROTEIN 10g; CARB 12g; FIBER 3g; CHOL 146mg; IRON 2mg; SODIUM 534mg; CALC 88mg

Baked Eggs with Chopped Tomato and Chives

These eggs are easy enough to prepare on busy mornings yet special enough to serve to guests at your next brunch. Round out the meal with fresh strawberries.

Butter-flavored cooking spray
2   **medium tomatoes, seeded and chopped**
2   **tablespoons minced fresh chives**
4   **large eggs**
½   **teaspoon salt**
½   **teaspoon freshly ground black pepper**

1. Preheat oven to 375°.
2. Coat 4 (4-ounce) ramekins or custard cups with cooking spray. Spoon tomato and chives evenly into each ramekin. Break 1 egg on top of tomato mixture in each ramekin; sprinkle evenly with salt and pepper.
3. Bake at 375° for 13 minutes or until desired degree of doneness.

YIELD | SERVES 4 (SERVING SIZE: 1 RAMEKIN)

CALORIES 87; FAT 5.5g (sat 1.6g, mono 1.8g, poly 0.9g); PROTEIN 7g; CARB 3g; FIBER 1g; CHOL 212mg; IRON 1mg; SODIUM 364mg; CALC 35mg

Baked Eggs with Kale Sauté

Baked eggs sit atop a nest of sweet potato and kale hash for this creative brunch entrée. Adjust the baking time depending on how well done you like your eggs.

- 2 teaspoons olive oil
- 1 cup chopped onion
- 2 garlic cloves, minced
- 1 large peeled sweet potato (about 1 pound), cut into 1 x 2-inch cubes
- ¾ cup fat-free, lower-sodium chicken broth
- 6 cups chopped kale
- ½ teaspoon hot smoked paprika
- ¼ teaspoon salt, divided
- ¼ teaspoon freshly ground black pepper, divided
- 4 large eggs
- Additional hot smoked paprika (optional)

1. Preheat oven to 350°.

2. Heat oil in a large ovenproof nonstick skillet over medium-high heat. Add onion to pan; sauté 4 minutes or until tender. Add garlic; sauté 30 seconds. Add sweet potato; cook 6 minutes or until potato is golden brown, stirring occasionally. Stir in broth; bring to a boil. Cover, reduce heat, and simmer 5 minutes or until sweet potato is almost tender. Increase heat to medium-high. Add kale; cook, uncovered, 4 minutes or until kale wilts, stirring occasionally. Stir in ½ teaspoon paprika, ⅛ teaspoon salt, and ⅛ teaspoon pepper; remove pan from heat.

3. Break eggs, 1 at a time, on top of kale mixture; sprinkle with remaining ⅛ teaspoon salt and remaining ⅛ teaspoon pepper.

4. Bake at 350° for 8 to 10 minutes or until eggs are desired degree of doneness. Sprinkle with additional paprika, if desired.

YIELD | SERVES 4 (SERVING SIZE: ¼ OF KALE MIXTURE AND 1 EGG)

CALORIES 280; FAT 9.9g (sat 3.2g, mono 3.9g, poly 1.6g); PROTEIN 16g; CARB 34g; FIBER 7g; CHOL 190mg; IRON 3mg; SODIUM 623mg; CALC 251mg

Baked Eggs with Canadian Bacon

Cooking spray
6 (1-ounce) slices Canadian bacon
¾ teaspoon hot sauce
6 large eggs
⅛ teaspoon salt
⅛ teaspoon freshly ground black pepper

1. Preheat oven to 350°.
2. Coat 6 muffin cups with cooking spray, and place 1 Canadian bacon slice in each muffin cup. Top evenly with hot sauce. Crack 1 egg over hot sauce in each muffin cup; sprinkle with salt and pepper.
3. Bake at 350° for 20 minutes or until set.

YIELD | SERVES 6 (SERVING SIZE: 1 EGG)

CALORIES 126; FAT 6.5g (sat 2.1g, mono 2.8g, poly 1.4g); PROTEIN 13g; CARB 2g; FIBER 0g; CHOL 196mg; IRON 1mg; SODIUM 540mg; CALC 45mg

Turkey Breakfast Sausage

1 pound ground turkey breast
¾ cup diced unpeeled pear
¾ cup finely chopped red bell pepper
½ cup finely chopped red onion
¼ cup chopped fresh cilantro
1 teaspoon dried rubbed sage
½ teaspoon salt
½ teaspoon ground cumin
½ teaspoon ground allspice
½ teaspoon crushed red pepper
1 tablespoon canola oil, divided

1. Combine first 10 ingredients in a medium bowl. Shape into 8 (½-inch-thick) patties. Heat 1½ teaspoons oil in a large nonstick skillet over medium heat. Add 4 patties; cook 4 minutes. Turn patties over, and cook 3 minutes or until done.
2. Remove patties from pan; drain on paper towels. Repeat procedure with remaining oil and remaining patties.

YIELD | SERVES 4 (SERVING SIZE: 2 PATTIES)

CALORIES 192; FAT 5.3g (sat 0.8g, mono 2.5g, poly 1.5g); PROTEIN 27g; CARB 9g; FIBER 2g; CHOL 46mg; IRON 1mg; SODIUM 375mg; CALC 18mg

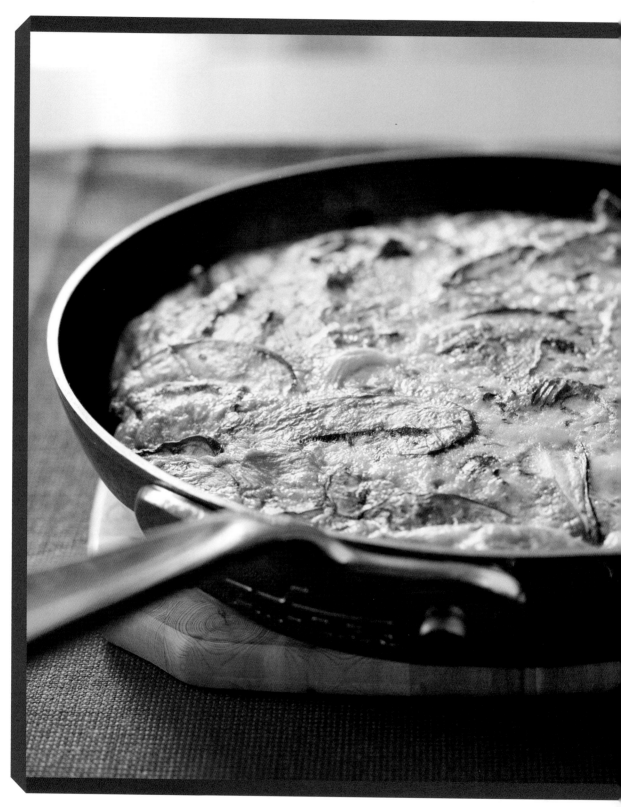

Mushroom Frittata

A frittata is a baked, open-faced omelet with Mediterranean flair.

- ¼ teaspoon freshly ground black pepper
- 8 large eggs
- ½ teaspoon salt, divided
- 1 tablespoon extra-virgin olive oil, divided
- 1 (8-ounce) package sliced mushrooms
- ¾ cup chopped green onions
- ⅓ cup chopped fresh basil
- 2 cups baby arugula
- 2 teaspoons lemon juice

1. Preheat oven to 350°.
2. Combine pepper and eggs; add ¼ teaspoon salt, stirring with a whisk. Heat a 10-inch ovenproof skillet over medium-high heat. Add 2 teaspoons oil; swirl to coat. Add mushrooms and remaining ¼ teaspoon salt; sauté 6 minutes or until mushrooms brown and most of liquid evaporates. Stir in onions; sauté 2 minutes. Reduce heat to medium. Add egg mixture and basil to pan, stirring gently to evenly distribute vegetable mixture; cook 5 minutes or until eggs are partially set. Place pan in oven. Bake at 350° for 7 minutes or until eggs are cooked through and top is lightly browned. Remove pan from oven; let stand 5 minutes. Run a spatula around edge and under frittata to loosen from pan; slide frittata onto a plate or cutting board.
3. Combine the remaining 1 teaspoon oil, arugula, and lemon juice. Cut the frittata into 6 wedges; top with arugula mixture.

YIELD | SERVES 6 (SERVING SIZE: 1 FRITTATA WEDGE AND ABOUT ⅓ CUP ARUGULA MIXTURE)

CALORIES 145; FAT 8.7g (sat 2.5g, mono 4.2g, poly 1.3g); PROTEIN 10g; CARB 4g; FIBER 0g; CHOL 243mg; IRON 2mg; SODIUM 352mg; CALC 87mg

Summer Vegetable Frittata

Garden-fresh summer vegetables will make this frittata a special breakfast or brunch treat.

- 1½ tablespoons olive oil
- 1 cup diced zucchini
- ½ cup chopped red bell pepper
- ⅓ cup chopped onion
- 1 tablespoon chopped fresh thyme
- ½ teaspoon salt, divided
- ¼ teaspoon freshly ground black pepper, divided
- 2 garlic cloves, minced
- ½ cup chopped, seeded tomato
- 9 large eggs

1. Heat olive oil in a 10-inch nonstick broiler-proof skillet over medium heat. Add zucchini, bell pepper, onion, thyme, ¼ teaspoon salt, ⅛ teaspoon black pepper, and garlic. Cover and cook 7 minutes or until vegetables are tender, stirring occasionally. Stir in tomato. Cook, uncovered, for 5 minutes or until liquid evaporates.
2. Combine eggs, remaining ¼ teaspoon salt, and remaining ⅛ teaspoon black pepper in a medium bowl; stir with a whisk until frothy. Pour egg mixture into pan over vegetables, stirring gently. Cover, reduce heat, and cook 15 minutes or until almost set in the center.
3. Preheat broiler.
4. Broil frittata 3 minutes or until set. Invert onto a serving platter; cut into 8 wedges.

YIELD | SERVES 4 (SERVING SIZE: 2 WEDGES)

CALORIES 227; FAT 16.4g (sat 4.2g, mono 8g, poly 2.1g); PROTEIN 15g; CARB 6g; FIBER 1g; CHOL 476mg; IRON 2mg; SODIUM 458mg; CALC 80mg

Prosciutto-Wrapped Melon Slices

Prosciutto (pro-SHOO-toh) is a salt-cured ham that is typically sliced thin and often eaten raw or lightly cooked. A little prosciutto offers a powerful punch of flavor in this dish, so you'll only need to use a small amount.

1   small cantaloupe, cut into 8 wedges
4   ounces thinly sliced prosciutto

1. Wrap melon slices evenly with prosciutto.

YIELD | SERVES 4 (SERVING SIZE: 2 WEDGES)

CALORIES 88; FAT 2.8g (sat 0.9g, mono 1.3g, poly 0.5g); PROTEIN 7g; CARB 9g; FIBER 0g; CHOL 17mg; IRON 1mg; SODIUM 443mg; CALC 12mg

SIMPLE SWAPS
Want a Variation?

Start your day with a solid blast of nutrients and protein. Omit the proscuitto, and serve hard-boiled eggs alongside the melon wedges. They're the ultimate, simple, on-the-go Paleo breakfast food.

Cantaloupe with Honey and Lime

Honey and lime juice add a burst of flavor to plain cantaloupe. This simple fruit dish is sure to brighten your breakfast any morning.

½	cantaloupe
4	teaspoons honey
4	teaspoons fresh lime juice

1. Cut cantaloupe into 4 wedges. Cut slits into each wedge, cutting into but not through rind. Drizzle each wedge with 1 teaspoon honey and 1 teaspoon lime juice. Serve immediately.

YIELD | SERVES 4 (SERVING SIZE: 1 WEDGE)

CALORIES 46; FAT 0.1g (sat 0g, mono 0g, poly 0.1g); PROTEIN 1g; CARB 12g; FIBER 1g; CHOL 0mg; IRON 0mg; SODIUM 11mg; CALC 7mg

Honey-Glazed Plums with Almonds

Honey helps the stone fruit caramelize lusciously on the grill.

- 3 **tablespoons honey**
- ½ **teaspoon chopped fresh thyme**
- ½ **teaspoon fresh lemon juice**
- 4 **large plums, pitted and halved**

Cooking spray

- 2 **tablespoons chopped toasted almonds**

1. Preheat grill to medium-high heat. Combine honey, thyme, and lemon juice in a large bowl. Add pitted and halved plums; toss gently to coat. Arrange plum halves, cut sides down, on grill rack coated with cooking spray; grill 3 minutes or until plums are well marked. Turn; grill 3 minutes or until tender. Arrange 2 plum halves on each of 4 plates; top each serving with 1½ teaspoons chopped toasted almonds.

YIELD | SERVES 4 (SERVING SIZE: 2 PLUM HALVES)

CALORIES 95; FAT 1.6g (sat 0g, mono 0.9g, poly 0.4g); PROTEIN 1g; CARB 21g; FIBER 1g; CHOL 0mg; IRON 0mg; SODIUM 0mg; CALC 13mg

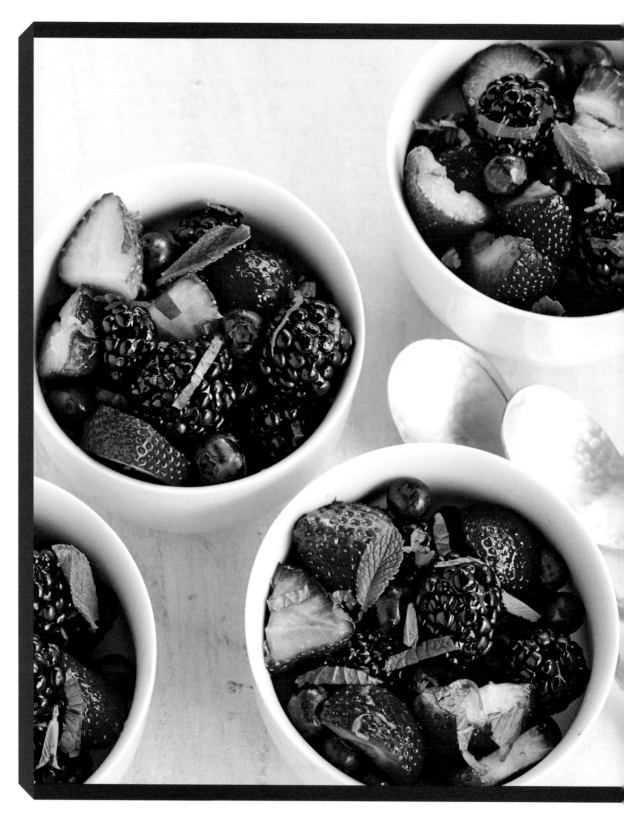

Berry-Ginger Salad

Use a combination of your favorite berries.

1	**tablespoon honey**
2	**teaspoons fresh lime juice**
½	**teaspoon grated peeled fresh ginger**
2	**cups mixed berries (such as blackberries, blueberries, and strawberries)**
1	**tablespoon chopped fresh mint**

1. Combine first 3 ingredients in a medium bowl. Add berries and mint; toss gently. Cover and chill at least 30 minutes.

YIELD | SERVES 4 (SERVING SIZE: ½ CUP)

CALORIES 50; FAT 0.3g (sat 0.0g, mono 0.0g, poly 0.2g); PROTEIN 1g; CARB 13g; FIBER 2g; CHOL 0mg; IRON 1mg; SODIUM 2mg; CALC 16mg

Blueberry Citrus Salad

Make this recipe ahead so you'll have a grab-and-go breakfast option on hand.

3	navel oranges
2	tablespoons chopped fresh mint
2	tablespoons honey
2	cups blueberries

1. Peel and section oranges over a bowl; squeeze membranes to extract juice. Stir in mint and honey. Add blueberries, and toss gently. Cover and chill 30 minutes.

YIELD | SERVES 4 (SERVING SIZE: ABOUT ⅔ CUP)

CALORIES 126; FAT 0.4g (sat 0g, mono 0.1g, poly 0.2g); PROTEIN 2g; CARB 33g; FIBER 4g; CHOL 0mg; IRON 0mg; SODIUM 3mg; CALC 52mg

Watermelon-Blueberry Salad

Toss this salad just before serving so the fruit doesn't water out and dilute the dressing.

4	cups cubed, seeded watermelon
½	cup blueberries
¼	cup honey
1½	tablespoons fresh lemon juice
1½	tablespoons olive oil
¼	teaspoon salt
⅛	teaspoon freshly ground black pepper
2	tablespoons chopped fresh mint

1. Place watermelon and blueberries in a medium bowl.
2. Combine honey and next 4 ingredients in a small bowl, stirring with a whisk. Stir in mint. Drizzle dressing over fruit; toss gently.

YIELD | SERVES 4 (SERVING SIZE: ABOUT 1 CUP)

CALORIES 168; FAT 5.6g (sat 0.8g, mono 3.8g, poly 0.9g); PROTEIN 1g; CARB 32g; FIBER 1g; CHOL 0mg; IRON 1mg; SODIUM 151mg; CALC 17mg

Raspberry-Banana Smoothie

The beautiful color of this quick smoothie makes a cheery treat.

1	small banana
1	cup frozen unsweetened raspberries
1	cup coconut milk
1	cup ice

1. Place all ingredients in a blender, and process until smooth. Serve immediately.

YIELD | SERVES 2 (SERVING SIZE: ABOUT ¾ CUP)

CALORIES 151; FAT 0.8g (sat 0.2g, mono 0g, poly 0g); PROTEIN 5.6g; CARB 32.4g; FIBER 4.2g; CHOL 2mg; IRON 0.5mg; SODIUM 63mg; CALC 174mg

Sunshine Smoothie

This slightly sweet, thick drink is a great snack or part of a breakfast: Just one serving offers about one-third of the day's vitamin C and vitamin A and about 10 percent of the potassium in a low-calorie package.

½   cup chopped, peeled mango
1½ cups chopped, peeled apricots (about 4 small)
⅔   cup chopped, peeled nectarine (about 1 medium)
1   cup chopped cantaloupe
⅛   teaspoon grated lemon rind
1   cup coconut milk
1   cup ice cubes

1. Place mango in a zip-top plastic bag; seal. Freeze 1 hour.
2. Combine chopped apricots and next 4 ingredients (through coconut milk) in a blender; process until smooth. Add frozen mango and ice; process until smooth.

YIELD | SERVES 4 (SERVING SIZE: ABOUT 1 CUP)

CALORIES 104; FAT 0.9g (sat 0.4g, mono 0.3g, poly 0.1g); PROTEIN 3g; CARB 23g; FIBER 3g; CHOL 2mg; IRON 0mg; SODIUM 36mg; CALC 86mg

SIMPLE SWAPS
Want Milk?

One of the easiest swaps when you switch to Paleo is coconut milk as a substitute for dairy milk. Choose the full-fat version: It tastes rich so you won't need much whether you're using it over fruit or in your coffee or tea. Another option is nondairy nut milks. You can find these in most stores, but check the ingredient list so you're not getting too much sugar or artificial additives.

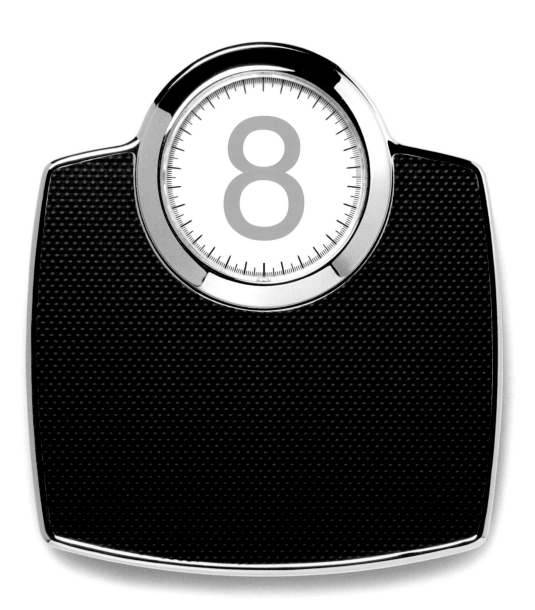

BUILD A BETTER LUNCH! Just as crucial as breakfast in terms of keeping you satisfied, your midday meal should help you power through your afternoon. With plenty of to-go options like protein-packed lettuce wraps, soups, and salads, you'll find a variety of options to mix up your brown bag repertoire.

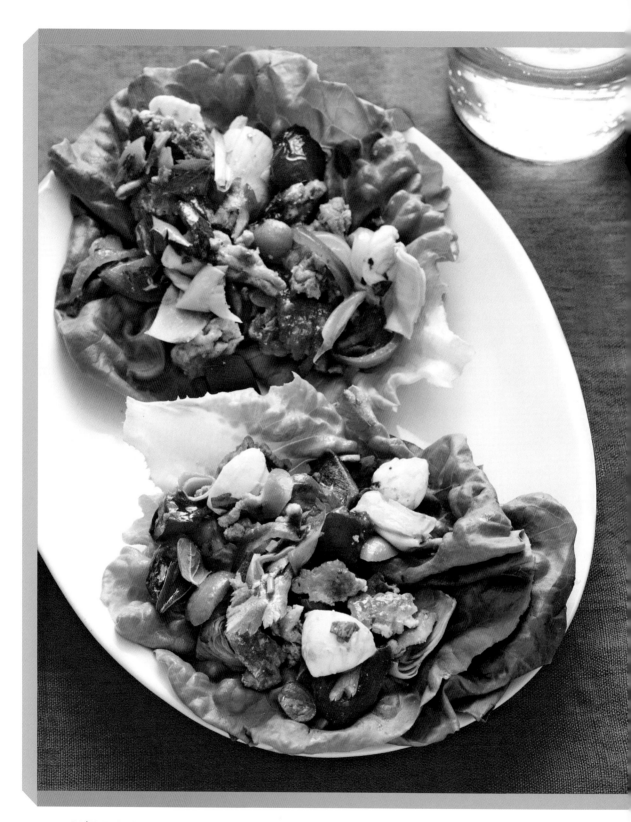

Chicken Lettuce Cups

The artichokes and olives amp up the flavor of this dish. To prep it even faster, toss the herbs, onion, artichokes, tomato, and olives in a food processor and pulse.

Cooking spray
- 1 **pound ground chicken**
- ¼ **teaspoon freshly ground black pepper**
- ⅛ **teaspoon salt**
- 1 **cup vertically sliced red onion**
- ¼ **cup canned artichoke hearts, drained and coarsely chopped**
- ¼ **cup diced tomato**
- 1 **tablespoon chopped fresh oregano**
- 1 **tablespoon chopped fresh flat-leaf parsley**
- 10 **pitted green olives, chopped**
- 1 **tablespoon fresh lemon juice**
- 8 **Bibb lettuce leaves**

1. Heat a large skillet over medium-high heat. Coat pan with cooking spray. Add chicken, pepper, and salt; cook 3 minutes, stirring to crumble.

2. Stir in onion and next 5 ingredients (through olives); cook 3 minutes or until chicken is done.

3. Stir in juice. Spoon 1¼ cups chicken mixture into each lettuce leaf.

YIELD | SERVES 4 (SERVING SIZE: 2 LETTUCE CUPS)

CALORIES 275; FAT 16.9g (sat 5.6g, mono 7g, poly 2.3g); PROTEIN 25g; CARB 7g; FIBER 1g; CHOL 115mg; IRON 2mg; SODIUM 495mg; CALC 27mg

Chicken and Mint Coleslaw Wraps

Fill up a cabbage leaf with this fresh and flavorful mixture of chicken, angel hair coleslaw, lemon juice, ginger, and mint for a simple sandwich meal.

4	(6-ounce) skinless, boneless chicken breast halves
⅛	teaspoon salt
	Cooking spray
⅓	cup fresh lemon juice
1	tablespoon fresh ginger (such as Spice World)
2	teaspoons agave
¼	teaspoon crushed red pepper
3	cups angel hair coleslaw
½	cup chopped fresh mint
1	poblano chile, halved lengthwise, seeded, and thinly sliced
6	large cabbage leaves

1. Place each chicken breast half between 2 sheets of heavy-duty plastic wrap; pound to ¼-inch thickness using a meat mallet or rolling pin. Sprinkle chicken with salt. Heat a large nonstick skillet coated with cooking spray over medium-high heat. Add chicken; sauté 4½ minutes on each side or until done. Remove chicken to a cutting board, and cut into thin strips.

2. Combine juice, ginger, agave, and red pepper in a large bowl. Add chicken strips, coleslaw, mint, and chile, tossing well to coat. Divide chicken mixture evenly among cabbage leaves; roll up.

YIELD | SERVES 6 (SERVING SIZE: 1 WRAP)

CALORIES 162; FAT 3.4g (sat 0.7g, mono 1.6g, poly 0.6g); PROTEIN 25g; CARB 6g; FIBER 2g; CHOL 37mg; IRON 2mg; SODIUM 206mg; CALC 37mg

Guacamole Chicken Wraps

Because of the generous amount of lime juice, the guacamole doesn't discolor.

2	tablespoons fresh lime juice
¼	teaspoon salt
1	ripe peeled avocado
½	cup chopped seeded plum tomato
4	green leaf lettuce leaves
2	cups shredded cooked chicken

1. Place first 3 ingredients in a medium bowl; mash with a fork until smooth. Stir in tomato.

2. Spread about ¼ cup avocado mixture on each lettuce leaf. Top each serving with ½ cup chicken. Roll up.

YIELD | SERVES 4 (SERVING SIZE: 1 WRAP)

CALORIES 175; FAT 7.5g (sat 1.4g, mono 4.2g, poly 1.2g); PROTEIN 23g; CARB 4g; FIBER 3g; CHOL 60mg; IRON 1mg; SODIUM 206mg; CALC 24mg

SIMPLE SWAPS

Mayo Makeover

Replacing the white stuff directly is tricky, so instead try using avocado. What your mouth and tongue are mostly looking for is a smooth, creamy texture to accompany your dish; avocado not only fits the bill, but it also surpasses mayo when it comes to flavor and health.

Beefy Jicama Wraps

Serve this plentiful wrap with a cup of fresh grapes for an easy supper. Look for jicama in the produce section of large supermarkets and in Mexican markets; choose roots that have thin skin (thick skin indicates that the jicama is old).

½   pound lean, boneless sirloin steak
½   teaspoon olive oil
⅛   teaspoon salt
½   teaspoon black pepper
1   cup (¼-inch) julienne-cut, peeled jicama (about ½ small jicama)
½   cup sliced red onion
1   tablespoon fresh lime juice
½   teaspoon chili powder
2   large lettuce leaves
¼   cup refrigerated fresh salsa

1. Cut steak across grain into very thin strips. Heat oil in a large nonstick skillet over medium-high heat. Add meat; sprinkle with salt and pepper. Cook 4 minutes or until meat is browned, turning occasionally.

2. Stir in jicama and next 3 ingredients (through chili powder); cook 2 minutes, stirring frequently.

3. Spoon filling evenly down center of each lettuce leaf. Roll up; serve immediately with salsa.

YIELD | SERVES 2 (SERVING SIZE: 1 WRAP AND 2 TABLESPOONS SALSA)

CALORIES 355; FAT 10.9g (sat 3.1g, mono 3.2g, poly 3.1g); PROTEIN 25g; CARB 37.2g; FIBER 6.8g; CHOL 55mg; IRON 5.1mg; SODIUM 631mg; CALC 121mg

Lamb Picadillo Wrap

If you prefer, substitute beef for lamb.

4	pounds boned lamb shoulder
2	tablespoons finely chopped seeded jalapeño pepper
1	tablespoon dried oregano
1	tablespoon chili powder
¼	teaspoon salt
3	garlic cloves, minced
1	(6-ounce) can tomato paste
2	cups water
½	cup golden raisins
¼	cup chopped pimento-stuffed olives
2	tablespoons minced fresh cilantro
2	tablespoons fresh lime juice
8	large lettuce leaves

1. Trim fat from lamb. Cut lamb into 3 x ¼-inch strips. Place a skillet over medium-high heat until hot. Add lamb; cook 4 minutes or until browned. Add jalapeño, oregano, chili powder, salt, and garlic, and sauté 1 minute. Stir in tomato paste, and sauté 2 minutes. Stir in 2 cups water and raisins; bring to a boil. Reduce heat; simmer 20 minutes. Stir in olives, cilantro, and juice.
2. Spoon about ½ cup lamb mixture down center of each lettuce leaf; roll up.

YIELD | SERVES 8 (SERVING SIZE: 1 WRAP)

CALORIES 320; FAT 10g (sat 3.7g, mono 4g, poly 1g); PROTEIN 25g; CARB 33g; FIBER 3g; CHOL 74mg; IRON 4mg; SODIUM 450mg; CALC 50mg

SIMPLE SWAPS
Lettuce Leaf Sandwiches

Let's face it: Sandwiches are mainly about what's inside, not the bread. So prepare your favorite fillers, and wrap them up. Romaine, chard, cabbage, or even iceberg lettuce leaves stand in nicely for bread or tortillas.

Tuna, Artichoke, and Roasted Red Pepper Wrap

A medley of Mediterranean flavors perks up humble albacore tuna in this no-cook dish. It can be made ahead for a lunch-to-go or prepared for dinner. Just add the spinach, and toss before serving.

1	(12-ounce) jar marinated, quartered artichoke hearts (such as Reese)
¼	cup chopped fresh dill
1	tablespoon olive oil
1	tablespoon fresh lemon juice
½	teaspoon freshly ground black pepper
2	garlic cloves, minced
2	cups chopped bagged fresh baby spinach
2	(5-ounce) cans albacore tuna in water, drained and flaked
1	(12-ounce) jar roasted red bell peppers, drained and chopped
4	large lettuce leaves

1. Drain artichokes, reserving 2 tablespoons marinade. Coarsely chop artichokes. Combine artichokes, reserved marinade, dill, and next 4 ingredients (through garlic) in a large bowl. Add spinach, tuna, and roasted peppers, tossing well.

2. Spoon mixture evenly into 4 lettuce leaves. Roll up.

YIELD | SERVES 4 (SERVING SIZE: 1 WRAP)

CALORIES 153; FAT 6.8g (sat 0.5g, mono 3g, poly 2.7g); PROTEIN 15g; CARB 9g; FIBER 2g; CHOL 23mg; IRON 1mg; SODIUM 468mg; CALC 17mg

Cajun Chicken Stew

Fresh okra is a Southern summer staple. Substitute frozen cut okra when fresh is not available.

1   teaspoon olive oil
2   cups sliced okra (about ½ pound)
1   (8-ounce) container refrigerated prechopped tomato, onion, and bell pepper mix
1½ teaspoons Cajun seasoning
3½ cups fat-free, lower-sodium chicken broth
2   cups shredded skinless, boneless rotisserie chicken breast

1. Heat oil in a Dutch oven over medium-high heat. Add okra and tomato mix; sauté 5 minutes or until vegetables are tender. Add seasoning, and cook 1 minute. Stir in broth and chicken; bring to a boil. Reduce heat, and simmer 10 minutes or until thoroughly heated, stirring occasionally.

YIELD | SERVES 6 (SERVING SIZE: 1 CUP)

CALORIES 115; FAT 2.5g (sat 0.6g, mono 1.1g, poly 0.5g); PROTEIN 17g; CARB 6g; FIBER 2g; CHOL 40mg; IRON 1mg; SODIUM 506mg; CALC 43mg

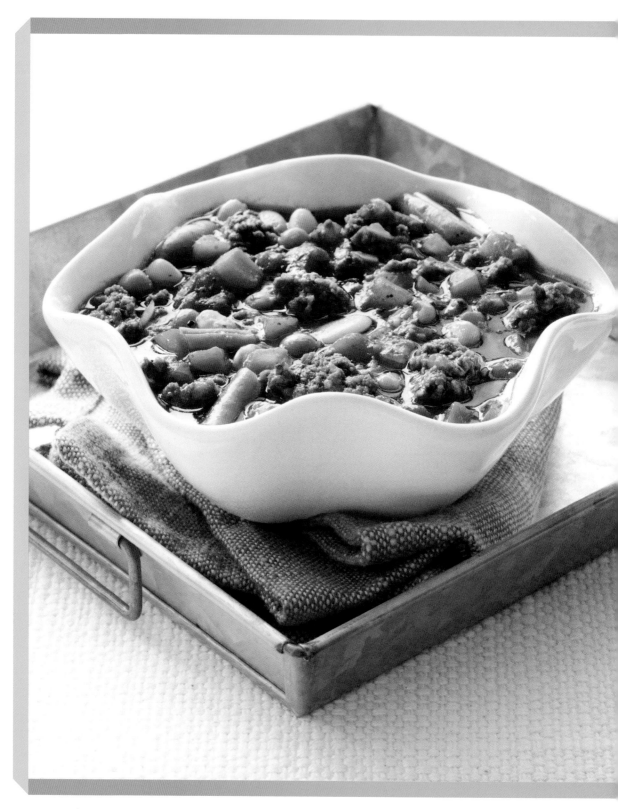

Easy Vegetable-Beef Soup

Italian-style stewed tomatoes and seasoning give this soup an Italian accent. Leftovers, if there are any, freeze beautifully.

1   (8-ounce) container refrigerated prechopped onion
1½   tablespoons minced garlic
1   teaspoon dried Italian seasoning
½   teaspoon black pepper
¼   teaspoon salt
1   pound ground round
2½   cups water
1   (16-ounce) package frozen mixed vegetables
1   (14½-ounce) can Italian-style stewed tomatoes, undrained and chopped
1   (8-ounce) can tomato sauce

1. Cook onion and next 5 ingredients (through beef) in a Dutch oven over medium-high heat until browned, stirring to crumble. Drain. Return meat mixture to pan. Stir in 2½ cups water and remaining ingredients. Bring to a boil over medium-high heat; reduce heat, cover, and simmer 20 minutes.

YIELD | SERVES 6 (SERVING SIZE: 1½ CUPS)

CALORIES 241; FAT 8.1g (sat 3.6g, mono 3.7g, poly 0.7g); PROTEIN 18g; CARB 21g; FIBER 4g; CHOL 49mg; IRON 3mg; SODIUM 514mg; CALC 63mg

Gazpacho with Lemon-Garlic Shrimp

Choose Pacific white shrimp farmed in fully recirculating systems or inland ponds.

1	(10-ounce) container grape tomatoes, divided
1½	cups sliced English cucumber, divided
1	cup diced red bell pepper, divided
¾	cup diced Vidalia or other sweet onion, divided
3	tablespoons extra-virgin olive oil, divided
2	tablespoons sherry vinegar
⅝	teaspoon kosher salt, divided
½	teaspoon freshly ground black pepper, divided
3	garlic cloves
1	(28-ounce) can San Marzano tomatoes, drained
1	tablespoon fresh lemon juice
1	teaspoon minced fresh garlic
20	medium shrimp, peeled and deveined (about 8 ounces)

1. Cut 8 grape tomatoes into quarters. Combine quartered tomatoes, ¼ cup cucumber, ¼ cup bell pepper, and ¼ cup onion in a small bowl; set aside.

2. Combine remaining grape tomatoes, remaining 1¼ cups cucumber, remaining ¾ cup bell pepper, remaining ½ cup onion, 2 tablespoons oil, vinegar, ½ teaspoon salt, ¼ teaspoon pepper, garlic cloves, and canned tomatoes in a food processor; pulse until almost smooth or until desired consistency. Refrigerate 25 minutes.

3. Combine remaining 1 tablespoon oil, juice, minced garlic, remaining ¼ teaspoon pepper, remaining ⅛ teaspoon salt, and shrimp in a medium bowl. Heat a large nonstick skillet over medium-high heat. Add shrimp mixture to pan; cook 3 minutes or until done, stirring occasionally.

4. Place about 1 cup soup into each of 4 bowls. Top each serving with 5 shrimp and ¼ cup cucumber mixture.

YIELD | SERVES 4

CALORIES 215; FAT 11.1g (sat 1.5g, mono 7.8g, poly 1.3g); PROTEIN 11g; CARB 19g; FIBER 5g; CHOL 71mg; IRON 2mg; SODIUM 587mg; CALC 111mg

Coconut Shrimp Soup

Light coconut milk adds subtle coconut flavor to this spicy soup. Use a vegetable peeler to remove the strips of rind from the lime, but be careful to avoid the white pith beneath because it can be very bitter.

1	cup light coconut milk
1	cup water
½	teaspoon red curry paste
¼	teaspoon salt
1	(2 x ½-inch) strip lime rind
¾	pound peeled, deveined large shrimp
¼	cup julienne-cut fresh basil

1. Combine first 5 ingredients in a large saucepan, stirring with a whisk. Bring to a boil over medium-high heat. Add shrimp; cover, reduce heat to medium, and cook 3 minutes or until shrimp turn pink. Remove and discard lime rind; stir in basil.

YIELD | SERVES 3 (SERVING SIZE: 1 CUP)

CALORIES 171 FAT 6.2g (sat 4.5g, mono 0.7g, poly 0.7g); PROTEIN 23.1g; CARB 4g; FIBER 0.1g; CHOL 172mg; IRON 2.8mg; SODIUM 441mg; CALC 65mg

Chicken and Lettuce Salad with Orange Dressing

To make this a brown-bag lunch, combine all ingredients except the lettuce; pack the lettuce and chicken mixture in separate containers, and combine right before serving.

1	large navel orange
3	tablespoons white wine vinegar
1	tablespoon olive oil
1	tablespoon honey
¼	teaspoon salt
⅛	teaspoon freshly ground black pepper
2	cup chopped chicken
1	(6.5-ounce) package sweet butter lettuce blend salad greens
¼	cup fresh mint leaves, torn

1. Peel and section orange over a large bowl, squeezing membranes to extract juice and placing sections in a separate bowl. Add vinegar and next 4 ingredients (through black pepper) to orange juice, stirring with a whisk. Add orange sections, chicken, lettuce, and mint; toss gently. Serve immediately.

YIELD | SERVES 4 (SERVING SIZE: 1¾ CUPS)

CALORIES 185; FAT 6.1g (sat 1.2g, mono 3.4g, poly 1g); PROTEIN 23g; CARB 11g; FIBER 2g; CHOL 60mg; IRON 1mg; SODIUM 206mg; CALC 30mg

Thai Seafood Salad

This flavorful main course salad is easy to whip up for lunch and can also be made ahead for a quick meal to grab on the go. Great fish sauce is essentially made with only water, salt, and fish, but be sure to check labels, as many bottles contain non-Paleo ingredients.

¼ cup water

8 ounces sea scallops

1 pound peeled, deveined medium shrimp

5 tablespoons fresh lime juice

2½ tablespoons fish sauce

1 teaspoon agave

1 teaspoon chile paste with garlic

1 cup red bell pepper strips

½ cup prechopped red onion

¼ cup fresh mint leaves, finely chopped

8 ounces lump crabmeat, drained and shell pieces removed

2 resh lemongrass stalks, trimmed and thinly sliced

1 cucumber, halved lengthwise and thinly sliced

1. Bring ¼ cup water to a simmer in a large skillet. Add scallops to pan; cover and cook 3 minutes or until done. Remove scallops from pan with a slotted spoon; pat scallops dry with paper towels. Place scallops in a large bowl. Add shrimp to simmering water in pan; cover and cook 3 minutes or until done. Drain well; add to scallops.

2. While scallops and shrimp cook, combine lime juice, fish sauce, agave, and chile paste.

3. Add juice mixture, bell pepper, and remaining ingredients to scallop mixture; toss gently to combine.

YIELD | SERVES 6 (SERVING SIZE: ABOUT 1⅓ CUPS)

CALORIES 180; FAT 2.4g (sat 0.4g, mono 0.3g, poly 0.9g); PROTEIN 31g; CARB 9g; FIBER 1g; CHOL 165mg; IRON 3mg; SODIUM 756mg; CALC 110mg

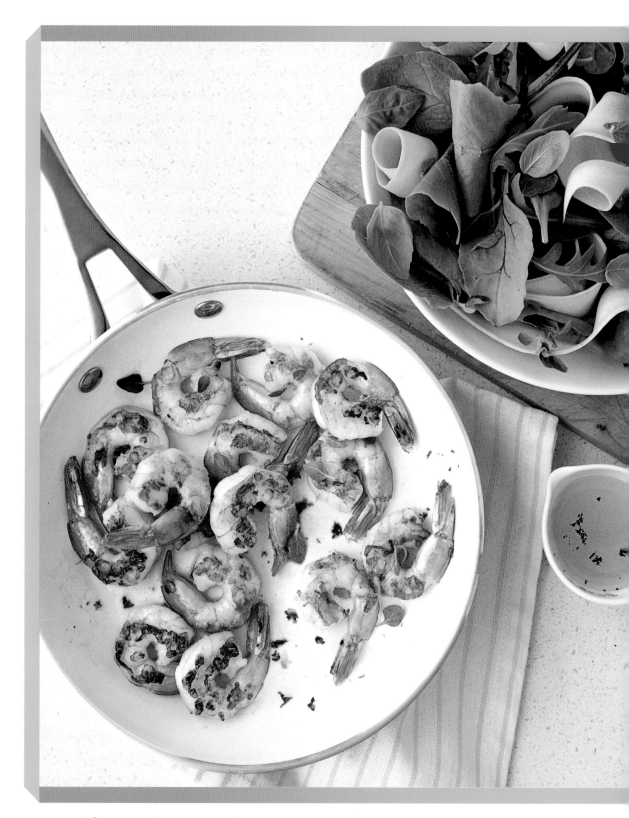

Shrimp and Herb Salad

Sustainable Choice: Choose U.S. Pacific white shrimp farmed in recirculating systems.

Cooking spray
1   pound peeled, deveined medium shrimp
⅜   teaspoon salt, divided
3   tablespoons olive oil
2   tablespoons fresh lemon juice
¼   teaspoon freshly ground black pepper
1   (5-ounce) package mixed salad greens (about 5 cups)
1   cup shaved yellow squash (about 2 medium)
¼   cup coarsely chopped fresh basil leaves
2   tablespoons coarsely chopped fresh oregano leaves

1. Heat a large skillet over medium-high heat. Coat pan with cooking spray. Sprinkle shrimp evenly with ⅛ teaspoon salt. Add shrimp to pan; cook 2 minutes on each side or until done.
2. Combine oil, juice, remaining ¼ teaspoon salt, and pepper in a medium bowl; stir with a whisk. Combine greens, squash, basil, and oregano in a large bowl. Add oil mixture; toss gently to coat. Divide salad mixture evenly among 4 plates; top with shrimp.

YIELD | SERVES 4 (SERVING SIZE: 1¼ CUPS SALAD AND ABOUT 3 OUNCES SHRIMP)

CALORIES 194; FAT 11.7g (sat 1.6g, mono 7.5g, poly 1.3g); PROTEIN 17g; CARB 6g; FIBER 2g; CHOL 143mg; IRON 1mg; SODIUM 417mg; CALC 81mg

Asian Tenderloin Salad

This salad has a nice balance of flavors. Grilled flank steak can substitute for the tenderloin, if you prefer.

1 pound beef tenderloin, trimmed
Cooking spray
3 tablespoons lime juice
2 tablespoons fish sauce
1 teaspoon honey
⅛ teaspoon ground red pepper
6 cups thinly sliced romaine lettuce
1 cup thinly sliced red onion
1 cup thinly sliced red bell pepper
1 cup thinly sliced peeled cucumber
⅓ cup coarsely chopped green onions
1 jalapeño pepper, seeded and minced
1 cup cilantro sprigs
¾ cup chopped fresh mint

1. Prepare grill.
2. Place beef on grill rack coated with cooking spray; grill 6 minutes on each side or until desired degree of doneness. Cover and let stand 10 minutes. Cut beef diagonally across grain into thin slices.
3. Combine juice, fish sauce, honey, and ground red pepper in a large bowl. Add beef, lettuce, and next 5 ingredients (through jalapeño); toss well. Add cilantro and mint; toss gently.

YIELD | SERVES 4 (SERVING SIZE: 1½ CUPS)

CALORIES 236; FAT 9.0g (sat 3.3g, mono 3.3g, poly 0.5g); PROTEIN 27g; CARB 12g; FIBER 4g; CHOL 71mg; IRON 5mg; SODIUM 717mg; CALC 66mg

Seared Steak Salad

Arugula, a peppery salad green, makes a tasty bed for tender,
simply seasoned pan-seared steak.

Cooking spray
4 (4-ounce) beef tenderloin steaks, trimmed
½ teaspoon salt, divided
¼ teaspoon black pepper, divided
2 teaspoons butter
½ cup prechopped red onion
1 (8-ounce) package presliced cremini mushrooms
2 tablespoons fresh lemon juice
2 cups grape tomatoes, halved
1 (5-ounce) bag baby arugula

1. Heat a large nonstick skillet over medium-high heat. Coat pan with cooking spray. Sprinkle
beef with ¼ teaspoon salt and ⅛ teaspoon pepper. Add beef to pan; cook 4 minutes on each
side or until desired degree of doneness. Remove beef from pan; keep warm.
2. Melt butter in pan; coat pan with cooking spray. Add remaining ¼ teaspoon salt, remaining
⅛ teaspoon pepper, red onion, and mushrooms to pan; sauté 4 minutes or until mushrooms
release their liquid. Combine juice, tomatoes, and arugula in a large bowl. Add mushroom
mixture to arugula mixture; toss gently to combine. Arrange 1½ cups salad mixture on each
of 4 plates; top each serving with 1 steak.

YIELD | SERVES 4

CALORIES 191; FAT 9g; (sat 3.8g; mono 3.1g; poly 0.5g); PROTEIN 21g; CARB 7g; FIBER 2g; CHOL 59mg; IRON 3mg;
SODIUM 349mg; CALC 72mg

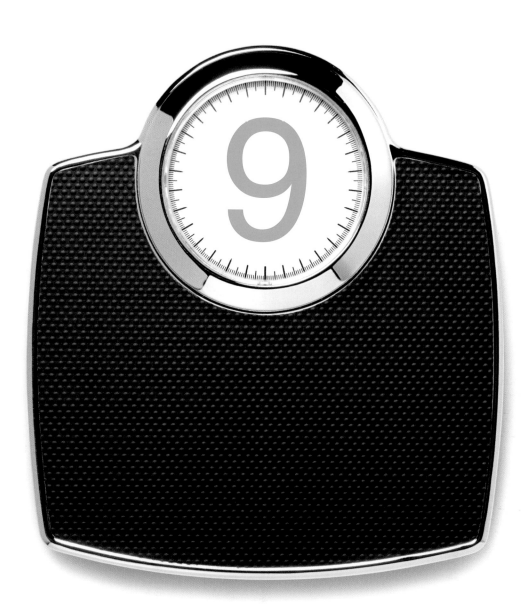

END YOUR DAY WITH an easy-to-prepare, home-cooked dinner. After a long, busy workday, you won't have to rely on take-out to get supper on the table quickly. Plan your evening meals around these incredibly flavorful poultry, fish, beef, pork, and lamb dishes—all guaranteed to satisfy.

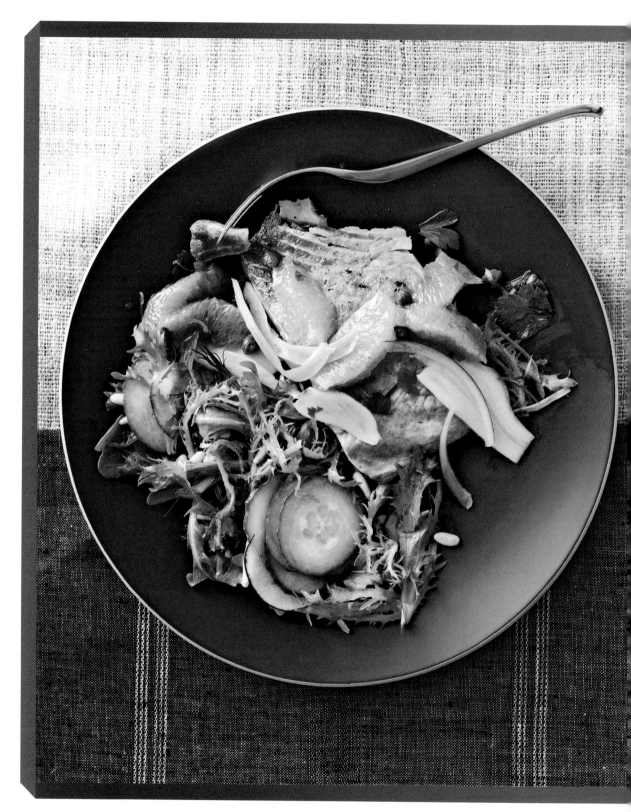

Arctic Char with Orange-Caper Relish

You can prepare the relish up to a day in advance. Pair the fish with a frisée and arugula salad, which you can prep while the fish cooks.

1	cup orange sections
2	tablespoons slivered red onion
1	tablespoon chopped fresh flat-leaf parsley
1	tablespoon minced capers
1	teaspoon grated orange rind
1	tablespoon fresh orange juice
1	tablespoon extra-virgin olive oil
1	teaspoon rice vinegar
⅛	teaspoon ground red pepper
4	(6-ounce) arctic char fillets
½	teaspoon kosher salt
½	teaspoon freshly ground black pepper
	Cooking spray

1. Combine first 9 ingredients in a small bowl. Cover and chill until ready to serve.

2. Heat a large heavy skillet over medium-high heat. Sprinkle fish with salt and black pepper. Coat pan with cooking spray.

3. Add fish to pan; cook 4 minutes on each side or until fish flakes easily when tested with a fork or until desired degree of doneness.

YIELD | SERVES 4 (SERVING SIZE: 1 FILLET AND ABOUT ¼ CUP RELISH)

CALORIES 295; FAT 18.5g (sat 2.9g, mono 7.7g, poly 2.4g); PROTEIN 27g; CARB 7g; FIBER 1g; CHOL 78mg; IRON 1mg; SODIUM 366mg; CALC 77mg

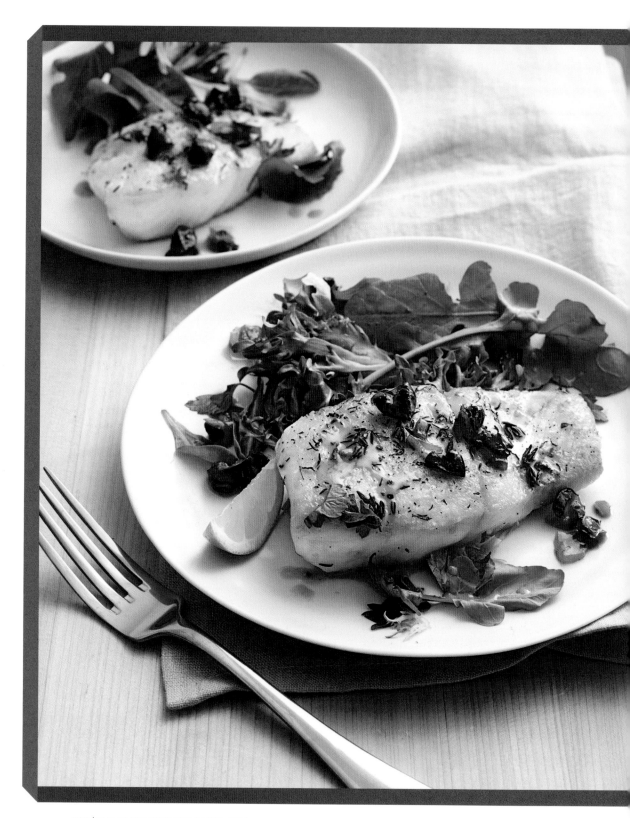

Halibut à la Provençal over Mixed Greens

Any type of packaged greens should work nicely in this recipe. Vary the mix of lettuces—baby arugula, spring mix, baby spinach— each time you make this. If you like, serve it with mashed sweet potatoes or cauliflower.

1   teaspoon dried herbes de Provence
2   tablespoons fresh lemon juice, divided
½   teaspoon salt, divided
4   (6-ounce) skinless halibut fillets
3   tablespoons olive oil, divided
½   teaspoon chopped fresh parsley
½   teaspoon chopped fresh thyme
¼   cup minced shallots
1   teaspoon honey
½   teaspoon Dijon mustard
¼   teaspoon freshly ground black pepper
2   tablespoons finely chopped pitted kalamata olives
1   (6-ounce) package mixed salad greens

1. Combine herbes de Provence, 2 teaspoons juice, and ¼ teaspoon salt. Rub over tops of fillets.

2. Heat a large skillet over medium-high heat. Add 2 teaspoons oil to pan; swirl to coat. Add fish to pan; cook 3 minutes on each side or until fish flakes easily when tested with a fork. Remove fish from pan; sprinkle with parsley and thyme.

3. Return pan to medium-high heat. Add remaining 7 teaspoons oil to pan; swirl to coat. Add shallots; sauté 2 minutes or until tender. Remove from heat; stir in remaining 4 teaspoons lemon juice, remaining ¼ teaspoon salt, honey, mustard, and pepper. Stir in olives. Combine greens and dressing in a bowl, tossing well.

YIELD | SERVES 4 (SERVING SIZE: 1 FILLET AND ABOUT 1½ CUPS MIXED GREENS)

CALORIES 308; FAT 15.6g (sat 2.2g, mono 9.8g, poly 2.5g); PROTEIN 35g; CARB 6g; FIBER 1g; CHOL 52mg; IRON 2mg; SODIUM 502mg; CALC 115mg

SIMPLE SWAPS

Missing Mashed Potatoes?

Sweet potatoes or cauliflower can mash up nicely yet still fit within a Paleo diet. Bake peeled sweet potatoes in foil, and then mash them while adding cinnamon and coconut oil or organic butter. For cauliflower, boil the cut-up florets for a few minutes until they're soft, thoroughly dry them, and then use your immersion blender (see Paleo Tools in Chapter 4) to mix them with organic butter. Add salt, pepper, garlic, scallions, and any other seasonings to taste.

Baked Citrus-Herb Salmon

Ask your fishmonger to remove the pin bones from the salmon. This dish is delicious served hot or at room temperature. It will feed a crowd, and you can toss the leftovers with mixed greens.

Cooking spray
1   (3½-pound) salmon fillet
1   teaspoon sea salt
½   teaspoon freshly ground black pepper
2   tablespoons grated lemon rind
1   tablespoon grated orange rind
10 fresh chives
4   thyme sprigs
4   oregano sprigs
4   tarragon sprigs
10 (⅛-inch-thick) slices lemon (about 1 lemon)

1. Preheat oven to 450°.
2. Line a shallow roasting pan with foil; coat foil with cooking spray.
3. Sprinkle fish with salt and pepper. Combine rinds; spread over fish. Arrange chives, thyme, oregano, and tarragon horizontally across fish. Arrange lemon slices on top of herbs.
4. Place fish on prepared pan. Cover with foil; seal. Bake at 450° for 30 minutes or until fish flakes easily when tested with a fork or until desired degree of doneness. Serve warm or at room temperature.

YIELD | SERVES 10 (SERVING SIZE: ABOUT 4 OUNCES)

CALORIES 213; FAT 9.8g (sat 2.3g, mono 4.3g, poly 2.3g); PROTEIN 29g; CARB 0g; FIBER 0g; CHOL 75mg; IRON 1mg; SODIUM 292mg; CALC 17mg

Pan-Seared Snapper with Garlic-Herb Vinaigrette

To prepare this easy fish recipe, simply sear the fish in a skillet, and then drizzle with a vinaigrette. Grouper or salmon would be a good substitute for the snapper.

2   tablespoons fresh lemon juice
1   tablespoon water
½   teaspoon salt, divided
½   teaspoon freshly ground black pepper, divided
1   garlic clove, minced
1½   tablespoons olive oil, divided
1   tablespoon minced fresh parsley
1   tablespoon minced fresh oregano
4   (6-ounce) snapper fillets
Cooking spray

1. Combine lemon juice, 1 tablespoon water, ¼ teaspoon salt, ¼ teaspoon pepper, and garlic in a small bowl; stir with a whisk. Gradually whisk in 1 tablespoon oil. Stir in parsley and oregano; set aside.

2. Sprinkle fillets with remaining ¼ teaspoon salt and remaining ¼ teaspoon pepper.

3. Heat remaining 1½ teaspoons oil in a large nonstick skillet coated with cooking spray over medium-high heat. Add fillets; cook 5 to 6 minutes on each side or until fish flakes easily when tested with a fork or until desired degree of doneness. Transfer fish to serving plates; drizzle with vinaigrette.

YIELD | SERVES 4 (SERVING SIZE: 1 FILLET AND 1 TABLESPOON VINAIGRETTE)

CALORIES 213; FAT 7.3g (sat 1.2g, mono 2.5g, poly 2.7g); PROTEIN 34g; CARB 1g; FIBER 0g; CHOL 60mg; IRON 0mg; SODIUM 369mg; CALC 60mg

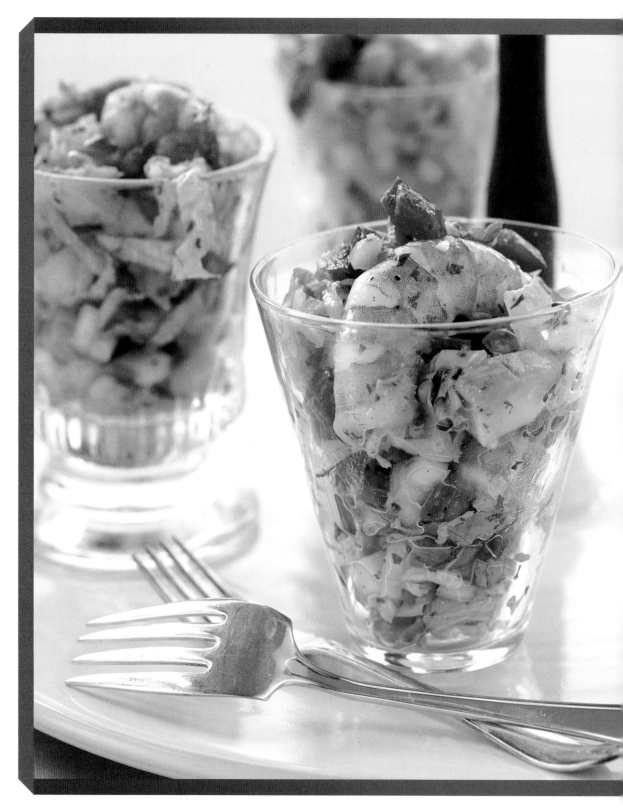

Spicy Shrimp and Avocado Salad with Mango Vinaigrette

For casual weeknight entertaining, try serving this salad in clear glasses instead of on traditional dining plates.

- ¼ cup fresh lime juice
- 2 tablespoons chopped fresh cilantro
- 1 tablespoon olive oil
- ½ teaspoon crushed red pepper
- ½ teaspoon coconut palm sugar
- ¼ teaspoon salt
- ¼ teaspoon freshly ground black pepper
- 1 garlic clove, minced
- ¾ cup diced mango (about 1 medium)
- 6 cups shredded romaine lettuce (2 hearts)
- 1 cup chopped red bell pepper (1 medium)
- 6 tablespoons thinly sliced green onions (optional)
- 1 pound peeled, cooked shrimp
- 1 avocado, diced

1. Combine first 8 ingredients in a large bowl, stirring with a whisk. Stir in mango. Add lettuce, bell pepper, and green onions, if desired; toss well. Add shrimp and avocado; toss gently.

YIELD | SERVES 4 (SERVING SIZE: 2¾ CUPS)

CALORIES 249; FAT 10.3g (sat 1.7g, mono 6g, poly 1.8g); PROTEIN 26g; CARB 15g; FIBER 5g; CHOL 221mg; IRON 5mg; SODIUM 412mg; CALC 86mg

Scallops with Tomato-Herb Broth

Naturally sweet scallops and pungent fresh herbs make this an impressive dish that takes just 10 minutes to cook.

1	pound sea scallops
2	garlic cloves, minced
2	teaspoons chopped fresh flat-leaf parsley
2	teaspoons chopped fresh basil
2	teaspoons chopped thyme
2	teaspoons chopped fresh oregano
¼	teaspoon salt
¼	teaspoon black pepper
2	large tomatoes, seeded and chopped (about 2 cups)
	Cooking spray

1. Rinse scallops; pat dry with paper towels. Set aside.

2. Combine garlic and next 7 ingredients (through tomatoes).

3. Coat scallops with cooking spray. Heat a large nonstick skillet over medium-high heat. Coat pan with cooking spray. Cook scallops in batches 2 minutes on each side or until browned. Add tomato mixture and scallops to pan, and cook 1 minute or until thoroughly heated.

YIELD | SERVES 3 (SERVING SIZE: ABOUT 6 SCALLOPS AND ½ CUP SAUCE)

CALORIES 160; FAT 1.5g (sat 0.2g, mono 0.5g, poly 0.5g); PROTEIN 27g; CARB 9g; FIBER 2g; CHOL 50mg; IRON 1mg; SODIUM 444 mg; CALC 61mg

Citrus-Herb Chicken

2	large limes
1	large ruby red grapefruit
1	large tangerine
1	large navel orange
¼	cup extra-virgin olive oil, divided
1	tablespoon minced garlic
1	tablespoon minced serrano chile
1	(3½-pound) whole chicken
¾	teaspoon kosher salt, divided
⅜	teaspoon freshly ground black pepper, divided
1	cup vertically sliced red onion
¼	cup chopped fresh mint
2	tablespoons chopped fresh cilantro

1. Grate 1 teaspoon rind and squeeze 5 tablespoons juice from limes. Place rind and 4 tablespoons juice in a medium bowl; place 1 tablespoon juice in a separate medium bowl. Grate 1 teaspoon grapefruit rind; section grapefruit. Grate 1 teaspoon tangerine rind; section tangerine. Grate 1 teaspoon orange rind; section orange. Add citrus sections to 1 tablespoon lime juice in bowl; set aside. Add grated rinds to lime rind mixture. Add 2 tablespoons oil, garlic, and chile to rind mixture; stir with a whisk.

2. Place chicken, breast side down, on a cutting board. Using poultry shears, cut along both sides of backbone, and open chicken like a book. Turn chicken breast side up; using the heel of your hand, press firmly against the breastbone until it cracks. Lift wing tips up and over back; tuck under chicken. Discard backbone and skin. Place chicken on a rimmed baking sheet. Spread citrus rind mixture over chicken. Cover and refrigerate at least 4 hours.

3. Position oven rack in lower third of oven. Preheat broiler to high.

4. Sprinkle chicken with ½ teaspoon salt and ¼ teaspoon black pepper. Broil chicken, breast side down, 20 minutes. Turn chicken over; broil an additional 20 minutes or until done, turning pan occasionally. Let stand 10 minutes.

5. Combine reserved citrus section mixture, remaining 2 tablespoons oil, remaining ¼ teaspoon salt, remaining ⅛ teaspoon pepper, red onion, mint, and cilantro; toss to combine. Serve with chicken.

YIELD | SERVES 4 (SERVING SIZE: ONE-FOURTH OF CHICKEN AND ½ CUP SALSA)

CALORIES 369; **FAT** 17.6g (sat 2.9g, mono 11.1g, poly 2.4g); **PROTEIN** 31g; **CARB** 24g; **FIBER** 7g; **CHOL** 92mg; **IRON** 3mg; **SODIUM** 473mg; **CALCIUM** 76mg

Italian-Seasoned Roast Chicken Breasts

Lean breast meat needs to be shielded as it cooks, so leave the skin on. Serve with sautéed spinach and mashed sweet potatoes for a hearty meal. Prepare them while the chicken bakes.

1	tablespoon chopped fresh rosemary
1	teaspoon grated lemon rind
2	tablespoons fresh lemon juice
4	teaspoons extra-virgin olive oil
½	teaspoon fennel seeds, crushed
½	teaspoon salt
½	teaspoon freshly ground black pepper
3	garlic cloves, minced
4	bone-in chicken breast halves (about 3 pounds)
	Cooking spray

1. Preheat oven to 425°. Combine first 8 ingredients in a bowl, stirring well.

2. Loosen skin from chicken by inserting fingers, gently pushing between skin and meat. Rub rosemary mixture under loosened skin over flesh; rub over top of skin.

3. Place chicken, bone side down, on a broiler pan coated with cooking spray. Coat skin lightly with cooking spray. Bake at 425° for 35 minutes or until a thermometer inserted into the thickest portion of the breast registers 155°. Remove chicken from pan; let stand 10 minutes.

YIELD | SERVES 4 (SERVING SIZE: 1 CHICKEN BREAST HALF)

CALORIES 240; FAT 12.2g (sat 2.8g, mono 6.3g, poly 2.1g); PROTEIN 30g; CARB 2g; FIBER 0g; CHOL 82mg; IRON 1mg; SODIUM 366mg; CALC 24mg

Chicken Kebabs and Nectarine Salsa

This company-worthy meal blends spice from the chicken with sweet and tangy nectarine salsa.

1	tablespoon coconut palm sugar
1	tablespoon olive oil
1	tablespoon fresh lime juice
2	teaspoons chili powder
1	teaspoon bottled minced garlic
½	teaspoon kosher salt
½	teaspoon ground cumin
¼	teaspoon freshly ground black pepper
1½	pounds skinless, boneless chicken breast, cut into 24 (2-inch) pieces
1	large red onion, cut into 32 (2-inch) pieces
	Cooking spray
2	cups diced nectarine (about 3)
½	cup diced red bell pepper
¼	cup thinly sliced red onion
2	tablespoons fresh cilantro leaves
1½	tablespoons fresh lime juice
2	teaspoons minced seeded jalapeño pepper
¼	teaspoon kosher salt
½	cup diced peeled avocado

1. Preheat broiler. Combine first 9 ingredients in a shallow dish; let stand 15 minutes.

2. Thread 4 onion pieces and 3 chicken pieces alternately onto each of 8 (12-inch) skewers. Place skewers on broiler pan coated with cooking spray. Broil 12 minutes or until chicken is done, turning occasionally.

3. Combine nectarine and next 6 ingredients (through ¼ teaspoon salt) in a bowl. Gently stir in avocado.

YIELD | SERVES 4 (SERVING SIZE: 2 SKEWERS AND ¾ CUP SALSA)

CALORIES 324; FAT 8.9g (sat 1.5g, mono 4.9g, poly 1.3g); PROTEIN 41g; CARB 19g; FIBER 4g; CHOL 99mg; IRON 2mg; SODIUM 547mg; CALC 44mg

SIMPLE SWAPS

Need Noodles?

Pasta can be sorely missed when you go Paleo. One nifty alternative is to use your spiralizer (see Paleo Tools in Chapter 4) and make noodles out of zucchini. They can be fried and mixed with pesto or tomato sauce for a satisfying pasta substitute.

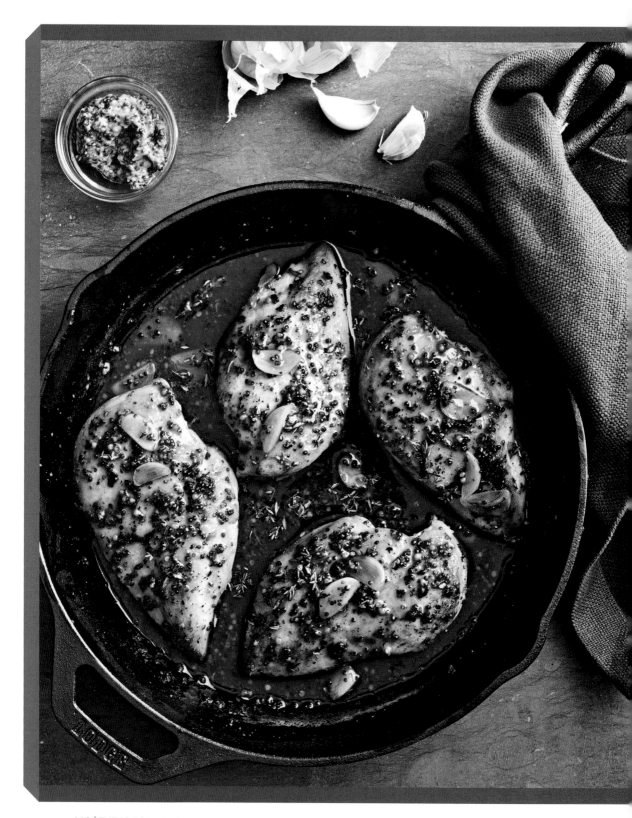

Maple-Mustard Glazed Chicken

The tangy-sweet flavor combination will work equally as well with chicken thighs or pork. Choose a cast-iron skillet to use for this recipe.

2	teaspoons olive oil
4	(6-ounce) skinless, boneless chicken breast halves
½	teaspoon freshly ground black pepper
¼	teaspoon salt
¼	cup fat-free, lower-sodium chicken broth
¼	cup maple syrup
2	teaspoons chopped fresh thyme
2	medium garlic cloves, thinly sliced
1	tablespoon cider vinegar
1	tablespoon stone-ground mustard

1. Preheat oven to 400°.
2. Heat a large ovenproof skillet over medium-high heat. Add oil to pan; swirl to coat. Sprinkle chicken with pepper and salt. Add chicken to pan; sauté 2 minutes on each side or until browned. Remove chicken from pan. Add broth, syrup, thyme, and garlic to pan; bring to a boil, scraping pan to loosen browned bits. Cook 2 minutes, stirring frequently. Add vinegar and mustard; cook 1 minute, stirring constantly.
3. Return chicken to pan; spoon mustard mixture over chicken. Bake at 400° for 10 minutes or until chicken is done. Remove chicken from pan; let stand 5 minutes. Place pan over medium heat; and cook mustard mixture 2 minutes or until liquid is syrupy. Serve with chicken.

YIELD | SERVES 4 (SERVING SIZE: 1 CHICKEN BREAST HALF AND ABOUT 1 TABLESPOON SAUCE)

CALORIES 264; FAT 4.4g (sat 0.9g, mono 2.2g, poly 0.7g); PROTEIN 40g; CARB 14g; FIBER 0.2g; CHOL 99mg; IRON 1.6mg; SODIUM 337mg; CALC 38mg

Spicy Herb-Rubbed Grilled Chicken

Place zucchini and red bell peppers next to the chicken on the grill for an easy and colorful side.

- **1   teaspoon onion powder**
- **1   teaspoon garlic powder**
- **1   teaspoon dried oregano**
- **½   teaspoon salt**
- **½   teaspoon cayenne pepper**
- **½   teaspoon freshly ground black pepper**
- **4   (6-ounce) skinless, boneless chicken breast halves**
- **Cooking spray**

1. Preheat grill to medium-high heat.

2. Combine first 6 ingredients in a small bowl. Sprinkle spice mixture over both sides of chicken, pressing lightly to adhere. Place chicken on grill rack coated with cooking spray; grill 6 minutes on each side or until done.

YIELD | SERVES 4 (SERVING SIZE: 1 CHICKEN BREAST HALF)

CALORIES 194; FAT 2.2g (sat 0.6g, mono 0.5g, poly 0.5g); PROTEIN 40g; CARB 2g; FIBER 0g; CHOL 99mg; IRON 1mg; SODIUM 406mg; CALC 27mg

Cilantro-Lime Chicken with Avocado Salsa

A three-minute dip into a pungent cilantro-lime marinade is all that's needed to deliver big flavor to chicken breasts.

Chicken:
2   **tablespoons minced fresh cilantro**
2½ **tablespoons fresh lime juice**
1½ **tablespoons olive oil**
4   **(6-ounce) skinless, boneless chicken breast halves**
¼   **teaspoon salt**
Cooking spray
Salsa:
1   **cup chopped plum tomato (about 2)**
2   **tablespoons finely chopped onion**
2   **teaspoons fresh lime juice**
¼   **teaspoon salt**
⅛   **teaspoon freshly ground black pepper**
1   **avocado, peeled and finely chopped**

1. To prepare chicken, combine first 4 ingredients in a large bowl; toss and let stand 3 minutes. Remove chicken from marinade; discard marinade. Sprinkle chicken with ¼ teaspoon salt. Heat a grill pan over medium-high heat. Coat pan with cooking spray. Add chicken to pan; cook 6 minutes on each side or until done.

2. To prepare salsa, combine tomato and next 4 ingredients (through pepper) in a medium bowl. Add avocado; stir gently to combine. Serve salsa over chicken.

YIELD | SERVES 4 (SERVING SIZE: 1 CHICKEN BREAST HALF AND ABOUT ¼ CUP SALSA)

CALORIES 289; FAT 13.2g; (sat 2.4g, mono 7.5g, poly 1.9g); PROTEIN 36g; CARB 7g; FIBER 4g; CHOL 94mg; IRON 2mg; SODIUM 383mg; CALC 29mg

Grilled Cumin Chicken with Tomatillo Sauce

Bring the heat of the Southwest to the dinner table with a delicious take on the weeknight meal of grilled chicken.

2	teaspoons olive oil
½	teaspoon ground cumin
⅛	teaspoon freshly ground black pepper
2	garlic cloves, minced
4	(6-ounce) skinless, boneless chicken breast halves
½	pound tomatillos
½	cup fat-free, less-sodium chicken broth
¼	cup cilantro leaves
¼	cup chopped green onions
2	tablespoons fresh lime juice
½	teaspoon coconut palm sugar
¼	teaspoon salt
1	garlic clove, chopped
1	jalapeño pepper, seeded and chopped
¼	teaspoon salt
	Cooking spray

1. Preheat grill to medium-high heat.

2. Combine first 4 ingredients in a large zip-top plastic bag. Add chicken to bag; seal and let stand 15 minutes.

3. Discard husks and stems from tomatillos. Combine tomatillos and broth in a small saucepan over medium-high heat; cover and cook 8 minutes. Drain and cool slightly. Combine tomatillos, cilantro, and next 6 ingredients (through jalapeño) in a food processor; process until smooth.

4. Remove chicken from bag; discard marinade. Sprinkle chicken with ¼ teaspoon salt. Place on grill rack coated with cooking spray; grill 6 minutes on each side or until chicken is done. Serve with tomatillo sauce.

YIELD | SERVES 4 (SERVING SIZE: 1 CHICKEN BREAST HALF AND ABOUT ⅓ CUP SAUCE)

CALORIES 237; FAT 5.1g (sat 1g, mono 2.3g, poly 1g); PROTEIN 40g; CARB 6g; FIBER 2g; CHOL 99mg; IRON 2mg; SODIUM 465mg; CALC 35mg

Chicken Thighs with Cilantro-Mint Chutney

For a refreshing side, sprinkle beefsteak tomato and cucumber slices with black pepper, and then drizzle with olive oil and lemon juice.

3 tablespoons grated fresh onion
½ teaspoon ground red pepper
10 garlic cloves, minced
2½ tablespoons olive oil, divided
2 teaspoons ground cumin, divided
4 (6-ounce) bone-in chicken thighs
½ teaspoon kosher salt, divided
Cooking spray
1 cup cilantro leaves
½ cup mint leaves
½ cup chopped green onions
2 teaspoons chopped, seeded jalapeño pepper

1. Combine first 3 ingredients in a large zip-top plastic bag; stir in 2 tablespoons oil and 1¾ teaspoons cumin. Add chicken to bag, seal, and massage marinade into chicken. Marinate in refrigerator 2 hours.

2. Preheat grill to medium-high heat.

3. Remove chicken from bag. Sprinkle chicken with ¼ teaspoon salt. Place on grill rack coated with cooking spray; grill 8 minutes on each side.

4. Combine cilantro, mint, onions, and jalapeño in a food processor. Add remaining 1½ teaspoons oil, remaining ¼ teaspoon cumin, and remaining ¼ teaspoon salt; process until smooth. Serve chicken topped with chutney.

YIELD | SERVES 4 (SERVING SIZE: 1 CHICKEN THIGH AND ABOUT 1½ TABLESPOONS CHUTNEY)

CALORIES 331; FAT 24g (sat 4.8g, mono 11.8g, poly 5.5g); PROTEIN 24g; CARB 5g; FIBER 1g; CHOL 135mg; IRON 2mg; SODIUM 332mg; CALC 4mg

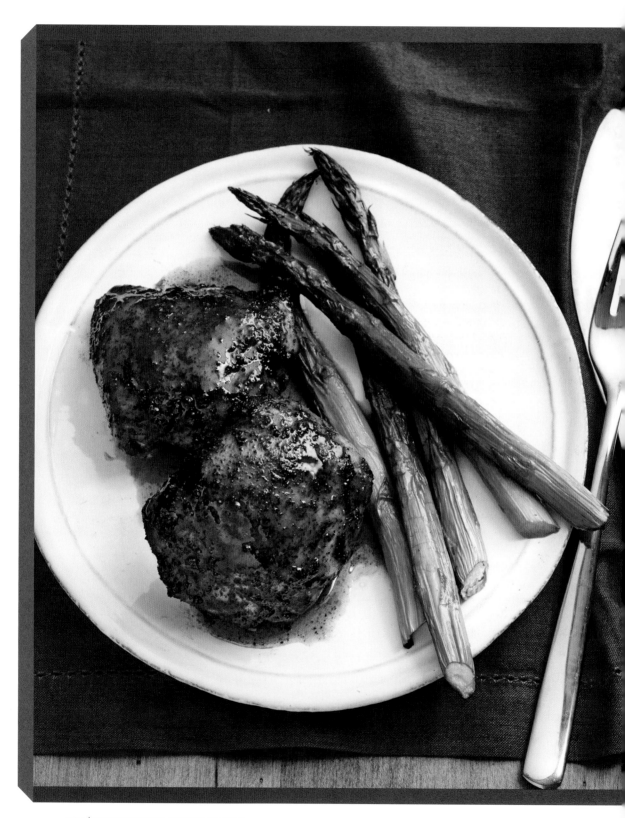

Spicy-Sweet Chicken Thighs with Roasted Asparagus

Once the chicken goes in the oven, trim and prep the asparagus on a separate baking sheet, and then place the pan in the oven when you turn the thighs over. Cook until asparagus is tender.

2	teaspoons garlic powder
2	teaspoons chili powder
1	teaspoon ground cumin
1	teaspoon paprika
½	teaspoon salt
½	teaspoon ground red pepper
8	skinless, boneless chicken thighs
	Cooking spray
1	pound asparagus, trimmed
1	tablespoon olive oil
6	tablespoons honey
2	teaspoons cider vinegar

1. Preheat broiler. Combine first 6 ingredients in a large bowl. Add chicken to bowl; toss to coat. Place chicken on a broiler pan coated with cooking spray. Broil chicken 5 minutes on each side.

2. While chicken cooks, combine asparagus and oil, tossing to coat. Spread asparagus in a single layer on a baking sheet, and broil 5 minutes or until tender.

3. While chicken and asparagus cook, combine honey and vinegar in a bowl, stirring well. Remove chicken from oven; brush ¼ cup honey mixture on chicken. Broil 1 minute. Remove chicken from oven, and turn over. Brush chicken with remaining honey mixture. Broil 1 minute or until chicken is done.

YIELD | SERVES 4 (SERVING SIZE: 2 CHICKEN THIGHS AND ABOUT 5 ASPARAGUS SPEARS)

CALORIES 363; FAT 14.5g (sat 3.5g, mono 6.6g, poly 2.9g); PROTEIN 30g; CARB 30g; FIBER 2g; CHOL 99mg; IRON 3mg; SODIUM 386mg; CALC 35mg

Chicken and Okra Stew

Look for okra pods between May and October, and choose ones that are firm, brightly colored, and short. Long okra pods tend to be tough. The "slime" that okra is known for will thicken this stew.

4	teaspoons olive oil, divided
2	pounds skinless, boneless chicken thighs, quartered
1	habanero pepper
1½	cups chopped green bell pepper
1	cup finely chopped onion
⅔	cup finely chopped celery
2½	cups chopped plum tomato
2	tablespoons chopped fresh parsley
1	tablespoon chopped fresh oregano
¾	teaspoon salt
1	teaspoon freshly ground black pepper
⅛	teaspoon ground cloves
1	(14-ounce) can fat-free, lower-sodium chicken broth
1	pound fresh okra pods, cut into 1-inch pieces

1. Heat 2 teaspoons oil in a Dutch oven over medium-high heat. Add half of chicken to pan; cook 6 minutes, browning on all sides. Remove chicken from pan. Add remaining chicken to pan; cook 6 minutes, browning on all sides. Remove chicken from pan.

2. Cut habanero in half. Seed one half of pepper, and leave seeds in other half. Mince both pepper halves. Add remaining 2 teaspoons oil to pan; swirl to coat. Add minced habanero, bell pepper, onion, and celery; sauté 5 minutes or until tender, stirring occasionally. Add tomato; cook 3 minutes or until tomato softens. Add parsley and next 5 ingredients; bring to a boil. Return chicken to pan; cover, reduce heat, and simmer 10 minutes. Add okra; cover and simmer 15 minutes or until okra is just tender.

YIELD | SERVES 4 (SERVING SIZE: 1⅓ CUPS STEW)

CALORIES 363; FAT 14.5g (sat 3.5g, mono 6.6g, poly 2.9g); PROTEIN 30g; CARB 30g; FIBER 2g; CHOL 99mg; IRON 3mg; SODIUM 386mg; CALC 35mg

Beef Chili

With ingredients like prechopped onion and less than 20 minutes cooking time, this flavorful chili comes together very quickly.

1	cup prechopped red onion
⅓	cup chopped, seeded poblano pepper (about 1)
1	teaspoon bottled minced garlic
1¼	pounds ground lean sirloin
1	tablespoon chili powder
2	tablespoons tomato paste
2	teaspoons dried oregano
1	teaspoon ground cumin
¼	teaspoon salt
¼	teaspoon black pepper
1	(14.5-ounce) can diced tomatoes, undrained
1	(14-ounce) can organic beef broth
½	cup chopped fresh cilantro
6	lime wedges

1. Heat a large saucepan over medium heat. Add first 4 ingredients; cook 6 minutes or until beef is done, stirring frequently to crumble. Stir in chili powder and next 7 ingredients (through broth); bring to a boil. Reduce heat, and simmer 10 minutes. Stir in cilantro. Serve with lime wedges.

YIELD | SERVES 6 (SERVING SIZE: ABOUT 1 CUP)

CALORIES 211; FAT 6.5g (sat 1.7g, mono 1.9g, poly 1.6g); PROTEIN 23g; CARB 16g; FIBER 5g; CHOL 54mg; IRON 3mg; SODIUM 474mg; CALC 52mg

Beef with Carrots and Dried Plums

1   (2½-pound) boneless chuck roast, trimmed
2   teaspoons sea salt
1   teaspoon freshly ground black pepper
2   teaspoons extra-virgin olive oil
3   cups thinly sliced onion
4   cups warm water
20 thyme sprigs
3   bay leaves
2   rosemary sprigs
1   sage sprig
1   pound baby carrots
2   cups pitted dried plums
    Sage leaves (optional)

1. Preheat oven to 350°.

2. Tie the roast at 2-inch intervals with twine; rub with salt and pepper. Heat oil in a Dutch oven over medium-high heat. Add roast; cook 12 minutes, browning on all sides. Remove roast from pan. Add onion and 4 cups warm water to pan, scraping pan to loosen browned bits. Return meat to pan.

3. Place thyme, bay leaves, rosemary, and sage on a double layer of cheesecloth. Gather edges of cheesecloth together; tie securely. Add cheesecloth bag to pan; cover, reduce heat, and simmer. Bake, covered, at 350° for 1½ hours. Turn roast; bake, covered, an additional 45 minutes. Add carrots and dried plums; bake, covered, an additional 45 minutes or until carrots are tender.

4. Place roast, carrots, and dried plums on platter; keep warm. Reserve cooking liquid. Discard cheesecloth.

5. Place a zip-top plastic bag inside a 2-cup glass measure. Pour reserved cooking liquid into bag; let stand 2 minutes (fat will rise to the top). Seal bag; carefully snip off 1 bottom corner of bag. Drain liquid into cup, stopping before fat layer reaches opening; discard fat. Slice roast; garnish with sage leaves, if desired. Serve with carrot mixture and sauce.

YIELD | SERVES 8 (SERVING SIZE: ABOUT 3 OUNCES BEEF, ½ CUP CARROT MIXTURE, AND ABOUT 1½ TABLE-SPOONS SAUCE)

CALORIES 316; FAT 9.4g (sat 3.2g, mono 4.4g, poly 0.5g); PROTEIN 31g; CARB 28g; FIBER 5g; CHOL 76mg; IRON 4mg; SODIUM 716mg; CALC 59mg

Steak Florentine

Traditionally, a thick-cut T-bone is the meat of choice for Steak Florentine, but we've substituted beef tenderloin steaks to significantly cut the fat. A paste of fresh garlic, rosemary, and olive oil infuses the steaks with flavor.

1 tablespoon olive oil
2½ teaspoons chopped fresh rosemary
4 garlic cloves, peeled
½ teaspoon freshly ground black pepper
¼ teaspoon salt
4 (4-ounce) lean beef tenderloin steaks (1½ inches thick), trimmed
Cooking spray
2 cups trimmed spinach
4 lemon wedges

1. Preheat grill to medium-high heat.
2. Place first 3 ingredients in a blender; process until mixture forms a paste, stopping blender and scraping down sides frequently.
3. Sprinkle pepper and salt over both sides of steaks; spread garlic paste over both sides of steaks.
4. Place steaks on grill rack coated with cooking spray, and grill 5 minutes on each side or until desired degree of doneness.
5. Divide spinach among plates; top with steaks. Squeeze a lemon wedge over each.

YIELD | SERVES 4 (SERVING SIZE: 1 STEAK AND ½ CUP SPINACH)

CALORIES 184; FAT 10.9g (sat 3.3g, mono 2.4g, poly 3.2g); PROTEIN 18g; CARB 2g; FIBER 0g; CHOL 54mg; IRON 2mg; SODIUM 186mg; CALC 32mg

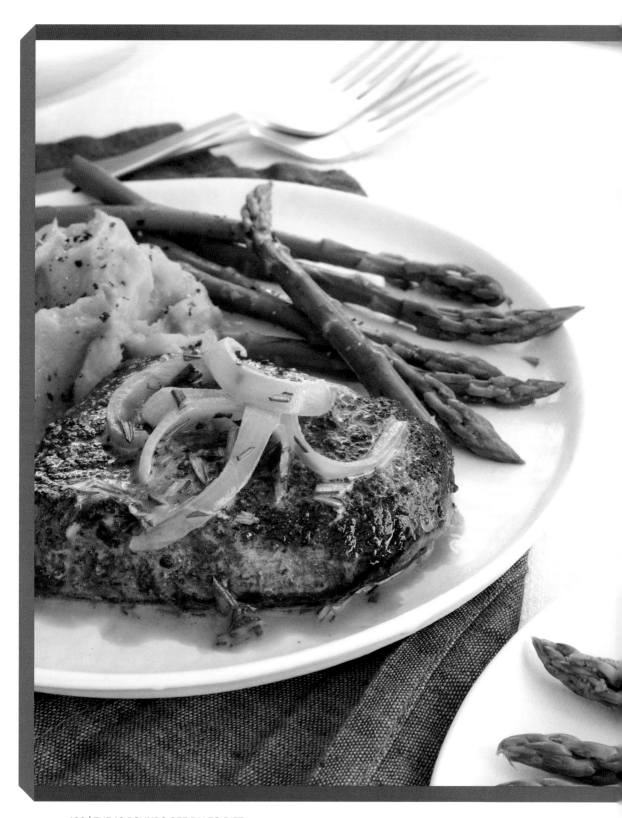

Beef Fillets with Rosemary Sauce

Accompany each fillet with steamed fresh asparagus and a half-cup mashed sweet potatoes for a complete meal.

4	(4-ounce) beef tenderloin steaks, trimmed (1 inch thick)
1	teaspoon freshly ground black pepper
½	teaspoon salt
	Cooking spray
½	small onion, sliced
½	cup fat-free, lower-sodium beef broth
1	teaspoon chopped fresh rosemary

1. Heat a large nonstick skillet over medium-high heat. Sprinkle steaks with pepper and salt; coat steaks with cooking spray. Add steaks to pan; cook 3 minutes on each side or until desired degree of doneness. Transfer steaks to a serving platter; keep warm.

2. Add onion to pan; sauté 30 seconds or until onion is tender. Add broth; cook 4 minutes or until liquid is reduced by half. Add rosemary; simmer 3 minutes or until slightly thick. Spoon sauce over steaks.

YIELD | SERVES 4 (SERVING SIZE: 1 STEAK AND 2 TABLESPOONS SAUCE)

CALORIES 196; FAT 5.6g (sat 2.1g, mono 2.2g, poly 0.2g); PROTEIN 25g; CARB 6g; FIBER 0g; CHOL 66mg; IRON 2mg; SODIUM 426mg; CALC 62mg

New York Strip with Carrots

Bacon lends the carrots a hit of smoky flavor.

- 2 (8-ounce) New York strip steaks, trimmed
- 2 teaspoons chopped fresh thyme
- 2 teaspoons chopped fresh oregano
- ½ teaspoon black pepper, divided
- ⅜ teaspoon salt, divided
- 3 teaspoons olive oil
- 1½ cups water
- 12 baby carrots, halved lengthwise
- 3 center-cut bacon slices
- Oregano leaves (optional)

1. Sprinkle steaks with thyme, oregano, ¼ teaspoon pepper, and ¼ teaspoon salt; press mixture into steaks. Heat oil in a large skillet over medium-high heat; swirl to coat. Add steaks to pan; cook 4 minutes on each side or until desired degree of doneness. Let stand 5 minutes; cut steaks across grain into thin slices.

2. Combine 1½ cups water and carrots in a large skillet over medium-high heat. Cover and bring to a boil. Cook 8 to 10 minutes or until carrots are tender. Remove carrots from pan. Wipe pan with a paper towel. Return pan to medium-high heat. Add bacon to pan; cook 4 minutes or until crisp. Remove bacon from pan with a slotted spoon; crumble. Add carrots to drippings in pan; sauté 3 minutes. Sprinkle with remaining ¼ teaspoon pepper, remaining ⅛ teaspoon salt, and crumbled bacon. Serve carrots with steak; garnish with oregano leaves, if desired.

YIELD | SERVES 4 (SERVING SIZE: 4 OUNCES STEAK AND ½ CUP CARROT MIXTURE)

CALORIES 306; FAT 17g (sat 7g, mono 6.7g, poly 0.9g); PROTEIN 29g; CARB 9g; FIBER 3g; CHOL 78mg; IRON 3mg; SODIUM 456mg; CALC 28mg

Steak and Avocado Kebabs

Give your barbecue a Southwest feel with these tasty Steak and Avocado Kebabs. The avocado's creaminess makes a pleasant texture contrast to the grilled beef on the kebabs. If using wooden skewers, soak them in water for 20 minutes before grilling so they don't burn.

1	teaspoon olive oil
¼	teaspoon kosher salt
½	teaspoon chipotle chile powder
¼	teaspoon black pepper
1	pound top sirloin steak
16	(1-inch) ripe avocado cubes
16	cherry tomatoes
16	(1-inch) squares red onion
8	(8-inch) skewers
	Cooking spray
¼	teaspoon kosher salt

1. Combine oil, ¼ teaspoon kosher salt, chipotle chile powder, and black pepper; rub over steak. Cut steak into 32 cubes. Thread steak, avocado, cherry tomatoes, and onion alternately onto skewers. Coat with cooking spray; sprinkle with ¼ teaspoon kosher salt. Place skewers on grill rack coated with cooking spray. Grill 5 minutes or until desired degree of doneness, turning skewers occasionally for an even char.

YIELD | SERVES 4 (SERVING SIZE: 2 SKEWERS)

CALORIES 226; FAT 11.3g (sat 2.6g, mono 7.0g, poly 1.0g); PROTEIN 24g; CARB 8g; FIBER 4g; CHOL 60mg; IRON 2mg; SODIUM 174mg; CALC 31mg

SIMPLE SWAPS

Rice Is Nice

And you can squeeze some in from time to time, depending on how closely you're following Paleo. But you may find that cauliflower rice gives you the taste and texture you crave with regular rice while remaining true to your Paleo plan. Chop up a head of cauliflower into florets, and pulse them in a food processor until they reach a rice-like consistency. If you sauté the results in ghee with onion, garlic, and pepper, you'll have some wonderful "rice" to complement your meal.

Beef Tenderloin with Chimichurri Sauce

Steak:

1   (15 x 6½ x ⅜–inch) oak grilling plank

4   (4-ounce) beef tenderloin steaks, trimmed (¾ inch thick)

¼   teaspoon salt

¼   teaspoon freshly ground black pepper

Sauce:

¾   cup fresh flat-leaf parsley leaves

¼   cup fresh cilantro leaves

¼   cup fresh mint leaves

¼   cup chopped onion

¼   cup fat-free, lower-sodium chicken broth

3   tablespoons sherry vinegar

2   tablespoons fresh oregano leaves

1   teaspoon olive oil

¼   teaspoon salt

½   teaspoon freshly ground black pepper

½   teaspoon crushed red pepper

3   garlic cloves

1. Immerse and soak plank in water 1 hour; drain.

2. Preheat grill, heating one side to medium and one side to high heat.

3. To prepare steak, sprinkle steaks with ¼ teaspoon salt and ¼ teaspoon black pepper. Place plank on grill rack over high heat; grill 5 minutes or until lightly charred. Carefully turn plank over; move to medium heat. Place steak on charred side of plank. Cover and grill 12 minutes or until desired degree of doneness.

4. To prepare sauce, combine parsley and next 11 ingredients (through garlic) in a food processor, and process until smooth. Serve with steaks.

YIELD | SERVES 4 (SERVING SIZE: 1 STEAK AND ¼ CUP SAUCE)

CALORIES 159; FAT 5.5g (sat 1.7g, mono 2.4g, poly 0.1g); PROTEIN 23g; CARB 6g; FIBER 1g; CHOL 60mg; IRON 4mg; SODIUM 677mg; CALC 52mg

Pork Medallions with Herbed Mushroom Sauce

Serve with roasted carrots for a complete meal.

1	**(1-pound) pork tenderloin, trimmed**
½	**teaspoon salt**
½	**teaspoon freshly ground black pepper**
1	**tablespoon olive oil**
1	**(8-ounce) package presliced cremini mushrooms**
1	**cup fat-free lower-sodium chicken broth**
1	**tablespoon chopped fresh thyme**
1	**tablespoon organic butter**

1. Cut pork crosswise into 12 slices; sprinkle pork with salt and pepper.

2. Heat oil in a large nonstick skillet over medium-high heat. Add pork to pan; cook 2 to 3 minutes on each side or until pork reaches desired degree of doneness. Remove pork from pan; keep warm.

3. Add mushrooms to pan; cook 3 minutes or until lightly browned, stirring occasionally. Stir in broth and thyme; cook until liquid is reduced to ½ cup (about 3 to 4 minutes). Stir in butter; cook 1 minute. Spoon mushroom sauce over pork before serving.

YIELD | SERVES 4 (SERVING SIZE: 3 PORK SLICES AND ABOUT ⅓ CUP MUSHROOM SAUCE)

CALORIES 210; FAT 10.5g (sat 3.4g, mono 4.5g, poly 1.8g); PROTEIN 26g; CARB 3g; FIBER 1g; CHOL 81mg; IRON 2mg; SODIUM 525mg; CALC 21mg

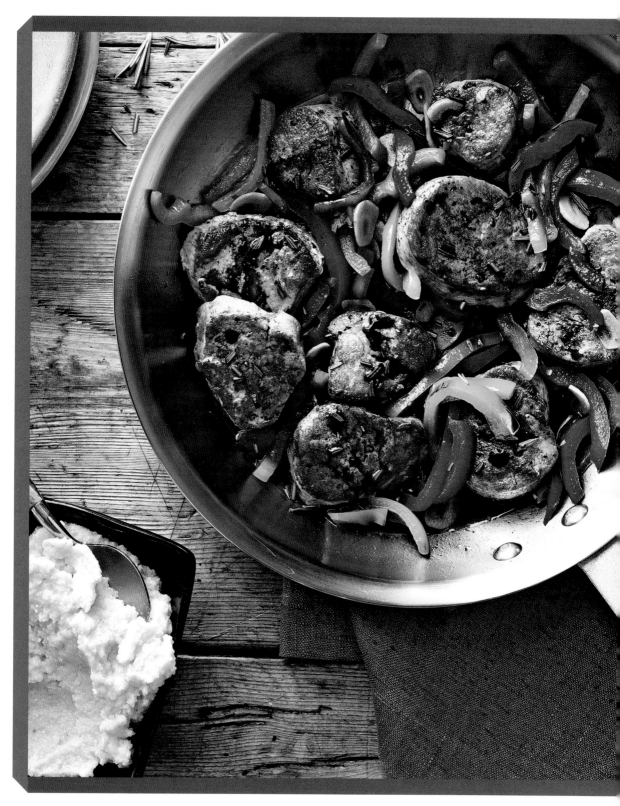

Pork Tenderloin with Red and Yellow Peppers

Don't let the anchovies scare you off; they add a depth of flavor that makes this dish taste like it took hours instead of just 20 minutes. Cutting the tenderloin into medallions means each bite is sure to have a bit of delicious seared crust.

1	(1-pound) pork tenderloin, trimmed and cut crosswise into 1-inch-thick medallions
½	teaspoon kosher salt
½	teaspoon freshly ground black pepper
1	tablespoon extra-virgin olive oil
1½	teaspoons chopped fresh rosemary, divided
4	canned anchovy fillets, drained and mashed
3	garlic cloves, thinly sliced
1	red bell pepper, cut into 1½-inch strips
1	yellow bell pepper, cut into 1½-inch strips
2	teaspoons balsamic vinegar

1. Heat a large skillet over medium-high heat. Sprinkle pork with salt and pepper. Add oil to pan; swirl to coat. Add pork to pan; cook 5 minutes.
2. Reduce heat to medium; turn pork over. Add 1 teaspoon rosemary, anchovies, garlic, and bell peppers; cook 7 minutes or until peppers are tender and pork reaches desired degree of doneness.
3. Drizzle pork with vinegar. Top with remaining ½ teaspoon rosemary.

YIELD | SERVES 4 (SERVING SIZE: 3 OUNCES PORK AND ABOUT ½ CUP BELL PEPPER MIXTURE)

CALORIES 215; FAT 10.1g (sat 2.7g, mono 5.4g, poly 1.2g); PROTEIN 25g; CARB 5g; FIBER 1g; CHOL 78mg; IRON 2mg; SODIUM 441mg; CALC 26mg

Spiced Pork Chops with Butternut Squash

Don't reserve pumpkin pie spice for desserts alone; sprinkle this blend of cinnamon, ginger, nutmeg, and allspice on pork chops for a fragrant, home-style dish.

Cooking spray

4　(4-ounce) boneless center-cut loin pork chops (about ¾ inch thick)

1　teaspoon pumpkin pie spice

½　teaspoon freshly ground black pepper

¼　teaspoon salt, divided

1　butternut squash (about 1¼ pound)

1　cup refrigerated prechopped onion

¼　cup water

1　tablespoon chopped fresh mint

1. Heat a large nonstick skillet over medium-high heat. Coat pan with cooking spray. Sprinkle pork evenly with spice, pepper, and ⅛ teaspoon salt. Add pork to pan; sauté 3 to 4 minutes on each side or until desired degree of doneness. Remove pork from pan; keep warm.

2. While pork cooks, pierce squash several times with a fork; place on paper towels in microwave oven. Microwave at HIGH 1 minute. Peel squash; cut in half lengthwise. Discard seeds and membrane. Coarsely chop squash.

3. Coat pan with cooking spray. Add squash; cover and cook 7 minutes, stirring occasionally. Add onion; cook, uncovered, 5 minutes, stirring frequently. Add ¼ cup water; cook until liquid evaporates, scraping pan to loosen browned bits. Remove from heat; stir in remaining ⅛ teaspoon salt and mint. Spoon squash mixture evenly over pork.

YIELD | SERVES 4 (SERVING SIZE: 1 PORK CHOP AND ¾ CUP SQUASH)

CALORIES 232; FAT 7g (sat 2.4g, mono 2.9g, poly 0.5g); PROTEIN 25g; CARB 18g; FIBER 3g; CHOL 65mg; IRON 2mg; SODIUM 200mg; CALC 96mg

Lemon-Herb Skillet Pork Chops

A squeeze of fresh lemon completes the dish and provides a hint of tartness that enhances the natural mild sweetness of the chops.

4	(4-ounce) boneless, center-cut loin pork chops (about ½ inch thick)
½	teaspoon salt
½	teaspoon black pepper
¾	teaspoon dried thyme
¾	teaspoon paprika
¼	teaspoon dried rubbed sage
1	tablespoon olive oil
4	lemon wedges

1. Sprinkle both sides of pork evenly with salt and pepper. Combine thyme, paprika, and sage. Sprinkle pork with herb mixture.

2. Heat oil in a large nonstick skillet over medium-high heat. Add pork; cook 4 minutes on each side or until pork reaches desired degree of doneness. Serve with lemon wedges.

YIELD | SERVES 4 (SERVING SIZE: 1 PORK CHOP AND 1 LEMON WEDGE)

CALORIES 218; FAT 10g (sat 2.9g, mono 5.4g, poly 1g); PROTEIN 25g; CARB 6g; FIBER 1g; CHOL 65mg; IRON 1mg; SODIUM 340mg; CALC 41mg

Slider Patties with Pomegranate Molasses

Here's an easy take on sliders that uses pomegranate molasses as a secret ingredient. It's available in Middle Eastern grocery stores and at large, well-stocked supermarkets. It is inexpensive and keeps well for a long time at room temperature.

- 1 pound lean ground lamb
- ¼ cup finely chopped fresh mint
- 2 tablespoons pomegranate molasses, divided
- ¾ teaspoon kosher salt
- ½ teaspoon ground coriander
- ¼ teaspoon ground red pepper
- ¼ teaspoon ground turmeric
- ¼ teaspoon ground cinnamon
- 1 garlic clove, minced

Cooking spray

1. Combine lamb, mint, 1 tablespoon pomegranate molasses, and next 6 ingredients (through garlic) in a large bowl. Divide mixture into 16 equal portions; gently shape each into a ¼-inch-thick patty.

2. Heat a grill pan over high heat. Coat pan with cooking spray. Add patties to pan; cook 1½ minutes on each side or until desired degree of doneness. Place patties on a platter; lightly brush patties with remaining 1 tablespoon pomegranate molasses.

YIELD | SERVES 4 (SERVING SIZE: 4 PATTIES)

CALORIES 282; FAT 15.2g (sat 6.3g, mono 6.4g, poly 1.1g); PROTEIN 19g; CARB 14g; FIBER 0g; CHOL 75mg; IRON 3mg; SODIUM 423mg; CALC 56mg

Rosemary Lamb Chops with Garlic-Balsamic Sauce

It's traditional in Rome to serve lamb for Easter, but these chops are too tasty and easy to wait for a holiday. From start to finish, they're ready in less than 30 minutes, making them ideal for busy weeknights.

- 2   tablespoons chopped fresh rosemary
- 2   tablespoons stone-ground mustard
- 1   tablespoon olive oil
- 1   tablespoon minced garlic, divided
- 2   teaspoons balsamic vinegar
- ½   teaspoon salt, divided
- 8   (4-ounce) lamb loin chops, trimmed
- ½   cup balsamic vinegar
- ½   teaspoon freshly ground black pepper

1. Preheat grill to medium-high heat.
2. Combine rosemary, mustard, olive oil, 1 teaspoon garlic, 2 teaspoons vinegar, and ¼ teaspoon salt in a small bowl; stir well with a whisk.
3. Place lamb chops in a shallow dish. Spread rosemary mixture over both sides of chops; let stand at room temperature 10 minutes.
4. While chops stand, bring ½ cup balsamic vinegar and remaining 2 teaspoons garlic to a boil in a small saucepan. Reduce heat, and simmer, uncovered, 5 minutes or until reduced to ¼ cup. Stir in remaining ¼ teaspoon salt and pepper; set aside, and keep warm.
5. Place lamb chops on grill rack; cover and grill 4 minutes on each side or until desired degree of doneness. Divide lamb chops among 4 plates, and drizzle with vinegar mixture.

YIELD | SERVES 4 (SERVING SIZE: 2 LAMB CHOPS AND 1 TABLESPOON SAUCE)

CALORIES 272; FAT 13.2g (sat 3.8g, mono 7g, poly 2g); PROTEIN 29g; CARB 6g; FIBER 0g; CHOL 90mg; IRON 2mg; SODIUM 480mg; CALC 31mg

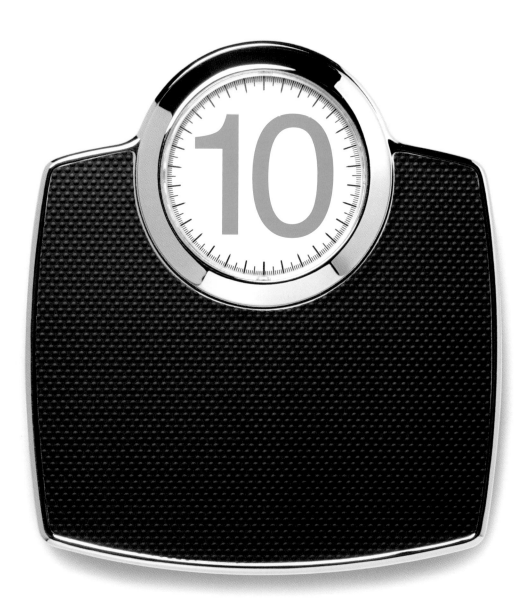

ANYONE WHO'S EVER TRIED to lose weight knows that snacks and side dishes can be a dieter's best friend. Whether they're salty, savory, crunchy, or creamy, they can help combat cravings and prevent hunger. Turn to these crisp salads, warm vegetables, crispy chips, and roasted seeds for rounding out meals and satisfying cravings.

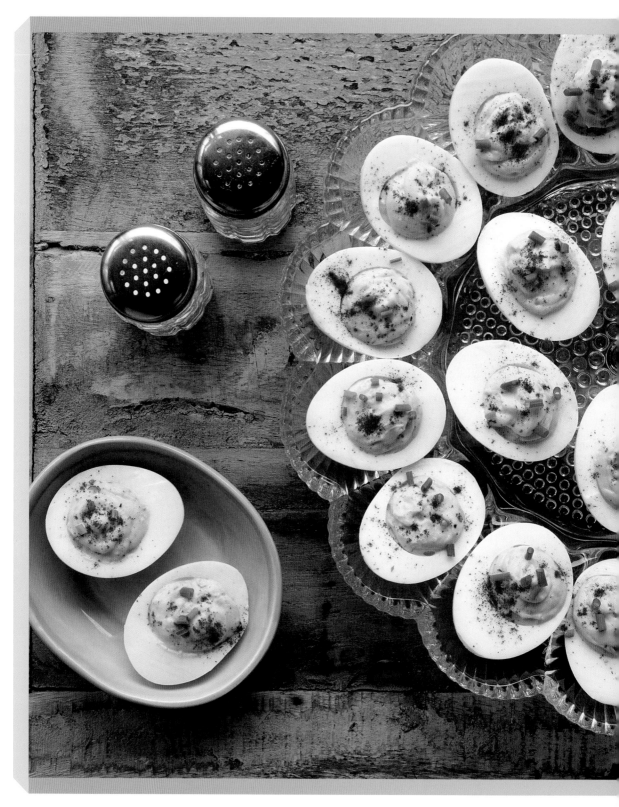

Deviled Eggs

To keep these portable snacks from turning on their sides when serving, use a deviled egg tray.

6	**large eggs**
3	**tablespoons olive-oil mayonnaise**
2	**teaspoons Dijon mustard**
½	**teaspoon fresh lemon juice**
¼	**teaspoon freshly ground black pepper**
2	**teaspoons coarsely chopped fresh chives**
⅛	**teaspoon hot paprika**

1. Place eggs in a large saucepan. Cover with water to 1 inch above eggs; bring just to a boil. Remove from heat; cover and let stand 15 minutes. Drain and rinse with cold running water until cool.

2. Peel eggs; cut in half lengthwise, and remove yolks. Place yolks in a bowl; mash with a fork. Stir in mayonnaise and next 3 ingredients (through pepper).

3. Spoon yolk mixture evenly into egg white halves. Sprinkle evenly with chives and paprika.

YIELD | SERVES 6 (SERVING SIZE: 2 EGG HALVES)

CALORIES 95; FAT 7g (sat 1.6g, mono 3.1g, poly 1.7g); PROTIEN 6g; CARB 1g; FIBER 0g; CHOL 186mg; IRON 1mg; SODIUM 129mg; CALC 29mg

Kale Chips

You'll never miss potato chips once you've had these. Cool the chips on the baking sheet so they'll crisp up even more after baking.

10½ ounces trimmed curly kale, torn into 2-inch pieces (about 14 cups)
1   tablespoon olive oil
¼   teaspoon kosher salt

1. Preheat oven to 350°.
2. Rinse kale; drain well, and pat dry with paper towels. Place in a large bowl. Drizzle with olive oil, and sprinkle with salt. Toss well. Place kale in a single layer on 3 (16 x 13–inch) baking sheets.
3. Bake at 350° for 15 minutes. (Watch closely to prevent leaves from burning.) Cool completely. Store in an airtight container.

YIELD | SERVES 4 (SERVING SIZE: 1 CUP)

CALORIES 67; FAT 4g (sat 0.5g, mono 2.5g, poly 0.6g); PROTEIN 2.5g; CARB 7.5g; FIBER 1.5g; CHOL 0mg; IRON 1.3mg; SODIUM 152mg; CALC 101mg

SIMPLE SWAPS

Power Popcorn

Here's another variation for versatile cauliflower: Set your oven to 450°. Trim the florets, and discard the core and thick stems of 1 head of cauliflower. Toss with olive oil and sea salt, and roast for about 45 minutes or until the pieces have turned golden brown.

Roasted Cauliflower and Sweet Peppers Skewers

Skewer roast cumin-coated cauliflower and peppers for a perfect Paleo party food.

3	tablespoons fresh lemon juice
1	tablespoon extra-virgin olive oil
1	teaspoon fine sea salt
1	teaspoon ground cumin
1	teaspoon ground coriander seeds
½	teaspoon cumin seeds
½	teaspoon crushed red pepper
30	cauliflower florets (about 1 medium head)
1	large yellow bell pepper, cut into 15 (1-inch) squares
1	large red bell pepper, cut into 15 (1-inch) squares
½	cup chopped fresh cilantro

1. Preheat oven to 450°.
2. Combine the first 7 ingredients in a large bowl, stirring with a whisk. Add cauliflower and bell pepper squares; toss gently to coat.
3. Spoon vegetables into a single layer on a jelly-roll pan. Bake at 450° for 25 minutes or until lightly browned and crisp-tender, stirring after 15 minutes. Cool completely; stir in cilantro.
4. Thread 1 cauliflower floret and 1 bell pepper square onto each of 30 (6-inch) skewers.

YIELD | SERVES 15 (SERVING SIZE: 2 SKEWERS)

CALORIES 25; FAT 1.1g (sat 0.1g, mono 0.7g, poly 0.1g); PROTEIN 1g; CARB 4g; FIBER 2g; CHOL 0mg; IRON 0mg; SODIUM 167mg; CALCIUM 15mg

Jicama with Red Chile and Lime

Peel this bulbous root vegetable with a knife rather than a vegetable peeler because the tough skin and outer layer are thick. Then slice, dice, or cut it into strips, and enjoy.

1	medium jicama (about 1 pound)
3	navel oranges, peeled, halved lengthwise, and cut crosswise into ¼-inch-thick slices (about 1½ cups)
2	small cucumbers, peeled, halved lengthwise, seeded, and thinly sliced (about 3 cups)
½	cup thinly sliced radishes
⅓	cup fresh lime juice
2	teaspoons dried ground guajillo chile or hot chili powder
½	teaspoon salt
⅓	cup coarsely chopped fresh cilantro

1. Peel and cut the jicama in half. Place halves cut sides down, and cut into ¼-inch-thick slices. Combine jicama, oranges, cucumbers, radishes, and juice in a bowl. Let stand 30 minutes. Add ground chile and salt, and toss well. Sprinkle with cilantro.

YIELD | SERVES 8 (SERVING SIZE: 1 CUP)

CALORIES 53; FAT 0.3g (sat 0.1g, mono 0g, poly 0.1g); PROTEIN 1g; CARB 12g; FIBER 5g; CHOL 0mg; IRON 1mg; SODIUM 153mg; CALCIUM 32mg

Masala Pumpkinseeds

This snack is made in a skillet using an Indian spice blend similar to curry powder called garam masala. The seeds double as a crunchy garnish for soups or salads.

½ teaspoon olive oil

1 cup raw pumpkinseeds (such as Woodstock Farms)

¾ teaspoon salt-free garam masala (such as Frontier)

¼ teaspoon kosher salt

¼ teaspoon ground cumin

Dash of ground red pepper

1. Heat a cast-iron skillet over medium heat until hot; add oil. Stir in pumpkinseeds.

2. Cook 4 minutes or until seeds are golden and begin to pop, stirring frequently. Cook, stirring constantly, 1 or 2 minutes or until most of the seeds are lightly browned. Remove from heat; stir in garam masala and remaining ingredients.

YIELD | SERVES 16 (SERVING SIZE: 1 TABLESPOON)

CALORIES 65; FAT 5.5g (sat 0.9g, mono 1g, poly 1g); PROTEIN 2.7g; CARB 1.4G; FIBER 0g; SUGAR 0g; CHOL 0g; IRON 1g; SODIUM 31g; CALC 1mg

SIMPLE SWAPS
Peanuts Gone to Seed

Who needs peanuts when you can have nutritious pumpkinseeds? Don't wait for Halloween to enjoy these treats: You can roast these year-round sprinkled with a variety of seasonings like garlic powder, onion powder, or just sea salt and pepper.

Trail Mix Poppers

Toss a few of these nutrient-packed poppers in a zip-top plastic bag, and you're ready to roll with treat in hand. Pair them with boiled eggs for a quick breakfast, too.

- ⅔   **cup sliced almonds**
- ¼   **cup flaked sweetened coconut**
- 1   **(7-ounce) bag dried fruit bits**
- 1½ **tablespoons honey**

1. Place almonds in a food processor; pulse 10 times or until minced. Transfer half of almonds to a medium bowl. Add coconut and fruit bits to remaining almonds in processor; process 30 seconds or until minced. Add honey. Pulse 10 times or just until blended.
2. Using a 1-inch scoop, shape mixture into 18 (1-inch) balls. Roll balls in reserved almonds. Store in an airtight container.

YIELD | 9 SERVINGS (SERVING SIZE: 2 POPPERS)

CALORIES 119; FAT 3.4g (sat 0.8g, mono 1.7g, poly 0.7g); PROTEIN 2g; CARB 21g; FIBER 3g; CHOL 0mg; IRON 1mg; SODIUM 18mg; CALC 26mg

Sweet and Spicy Snack Mix

This snack mix delivers a slight sweetness with a kick thanks to the ground red pepper.

Cooking spray
1½ teaspoons coconut oil
¼ cup honey
½ cup walnut halves
½ cup shelled pistachios
½ cup whole almonds
½ teaspoon ground red pepper
¼ teaspoon salt
¼ teaspoon ground cinnamon
1½ cups dried tart cherries

1. Line a baking sheet with foil; coat foil with cooking spray.
2. Heat coconut oil in a large nonstick skillet over medium-high heat. Stir in honey; cook 1 minute or until tiny bubbles form around edge of pan. Stir in walnuts and next 5 ingredients. Reduce heat to medium, and cook 5 minutes or until nuts are golden, stirring frequently. Stir in cherries. Immediately spread onto prepared baking sheet; cool completely.

YIELD | SERVES 15 (SERVING SIZE: ABOUT ¼ CUP)

CALORIES 145; FAT 7.2g (sat 0.9g, mono 2.9g, poly 3g); PROTEIN 3g; CARB 18g; FIBER 3g; CHOL 1mg; IRON 1mg; SODIUM 46mg; CALC 30mg

SIMPLE SWAPS

Mixed Trail Mix

Although it might seem like trail mixes would work with Paleo, most store-bought versions have too much milk chocolate, peanuts, and sugar to qualify. Make your own with almonds, walnuts, unsweetened dried fruit, and coconut shavings.

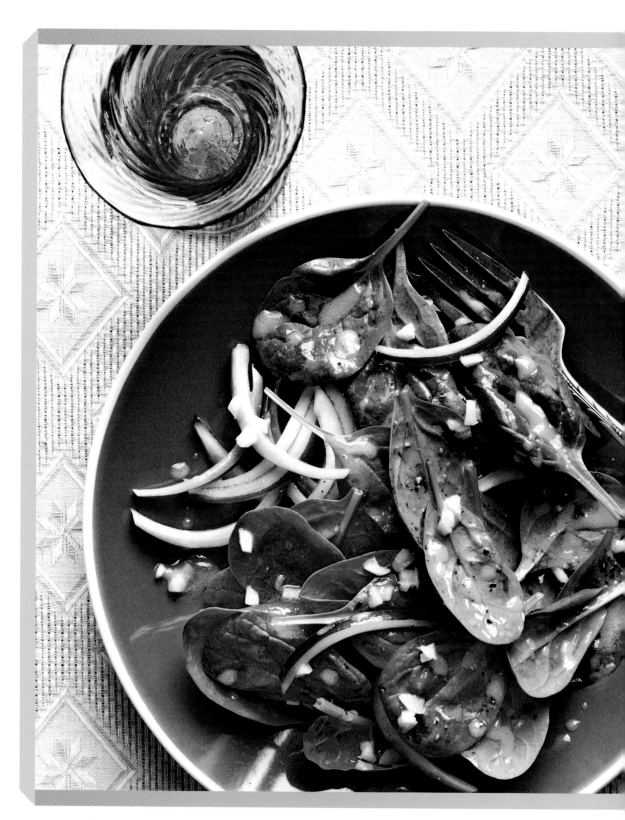

Spinach Salad with Garlic Vinaigrette

Baby spinach helps streamline prep since you won't spend time removing the stems.

1½	tablespoons extra-virgin olive oil
1	tablespoon white wine vinegar
½	teaspoon Dijon mustard
¼	teaspoon freshly ground black pepper
⅛	teaspoon salt
2	garlic cloves, minced
6	cups fresh baby spinach (about 6 ounces)
¼	cup vertically sliced red onions

1. Combine first 6 ingredients in a large bowl, stirring well with a whisk. Add spinach and onions; toss to coat.

YIELD | SERVES 4 (SERVING SIZE: 1¾ CUPS)

CALORIES 66; FAT 5.1g (sat 0.7g, mono 3.7g, poly 0.5g); PROTEIN 1.1g; CARB 5.2g; FIBER 1.9g; CHOL 0mg; IRON 1.3mg; SODIUM 147mg; CALC 31mg

SIMPLE SWAPS
Salad Dressing Stand-ins

Oil and vinegar are the perfect Paleo dressing, but beware of prepackaged versions that contain tons of sugar and preservatives and may not be made with olive oil. Whip up your own instead, and mix in pressed garlic, sea salt, and pepper to taste. Missing ranch dressing? Try a version with soaked raw cashews and coconut milk: Pulse ½ cup of the cashews in a food processor, and pulse until you get a paste, and then mix in a cup of coconut milk, some garlic and onion powder, lemon juice, sea salt, pepper, and dried dill.

Kale Salad with Pears and Walnuts

Both kale and walnuts are good sources of nutrients that are essential for a healthy diet. Kale is low in calories, high in fiber, and an excellent source of vitamins A, C, and K. Walnuts are a source of omega-3 fatty acids.

1	tablespoon sherry vinegar
2	teaspoons olive oil
1	teaspoon honey
⅛	teaspoon salt
⅛	teaspoon freshly ground black pepper
4	cups baby kale blend
1	Anjou pear, halved, cored, and cut crosswise into very thin slices
¼	cup chopped walnuts, toasted

1. Combine first 5 ingredients in a small bowl; stir with whisk. Combine kale and pear slices in a large bowl. Drizzle dressing over kale mixture, tossing to coat.
2. Divide kale mixture among 4 plates: sprinkle evenly with walnuts.

YIELD | SERVES 4 (SERVING SIZE: ¼ KALE MIXTURE, 1 TABLESPOON WALNUTS)

CALORIES 118; FAT 7.4g (sat 1g, mono 3.8g, poly 2.4g); PROTEIN 2g; CARB 12g; FIBER 3g; CHOL 0mg; IRON 1mg; SODIUM 117mg; CALC 86mg

Apple-Fennel Salad

If you can't find clementines, substitute two navel oranges.

  2   **tablespoons olive oil**
  2   **tablespoons white balsamic vinegar**
  1   **teaspoon honey**
 ¼   **teaspoon salt**
 ¼   **teaspoon freshly ground black pepper**
  2   **cups chopped Granny Smith apple (about 1)**
  2   **cups sliced fennel bulb (about 1 bulb)**
 ½   **cup sliced red onions**
  2   **cups chopped peeled clementines (about 4)**

1. Combine first 5 ingredients in a large bowl; stir with a whisk. Add apple, fennel, and onions; toss to coat. Add clementines, and toss gently. Cover and chill until ready to serve.

YIELD | SERVES 6 (SERVING SIZE: 1 CUP)

CALORIES 104; FAT 4.6g (sat 0.6g, mono 3.3g, poly 0.5g); PROTEIN 1g; CARB 16g; FIBER 3g; CHOL 0mg; IRON 0mg; SODIUM 116mg; CALC 33mg

Radish and Cilantro Slaw

Look for packages of angel hair slaw near the bagged lettuce at the supermarket. Pack any leftover slaw for lunch the next day.

3	cups packed angel hair slaw
½	cup chopped fresh cilantro
1	(6-ounce) bag radishes, trimmed and grated (about 1½ cups)
2	tablespoons fresh lime juice
1	tablespoon extra-virgin olive oil
1	tablespoon honey
½	teaspoon ground cumin
¼	teaspoon salt

1. Combine first 3 ingredients in a large bowl; toss well.

2. Combine lime juice and next 4 ingredients (through salt) in a small bowl; stir with a whisk. Pour dressing over slaw mixture; tossing gently to coat. Cover and chill until ready to serve.

YIELD | SERVES 4 (SERVING SIZE: ABOUT 1 CUP)

CALORIES 69; FAT 3.6 (sat 0.5, mono 2.7g, poly 0.3g); PROTEIN 0g; CARB 9g; FIBER 2g; CHOL 0mg; IRON 0mg; SODIUM 175mg; CALC 32mg

Lemon-Dill Carrot and Parsnip Hash

Sautéing grated carrot and parsnip enhances the slightly sweet flavors of these fiber-rich root vegetables. Pair this simple side dish with grilled chicken or fish.

2	teaspoons olive oil
½	pound carrots, peeled and grated (about 1½ cups)
½	pound parsnip, peeled and grated (about 1½ cups)
1	tablespoon chopped fresh dill
1	teaspoon grated fresh lemon rind
1	tablespoon fresh lemon juice
¼	teaspoon salt
¼	teaspoon freshly ground black pepper

1. Heat oil in a large nonstick skillet over medium-high heat. Add carrot and parsnip; sauté 5 minutes or until tender. Remove from heat; stir in dill and remaining ingredients.

YIELD | SERVES 4 (SERVING SIZE: ½ CUP)

CALORIES 87; FAT 2.6g (sat 0.4g, mono 1.7g, poly 0.3g); PROTEIN 1g; CARB 16g; FIBER 5g; CHOL 0mg; IRON 1mg; SODIUM 193mg; CALC 41mg

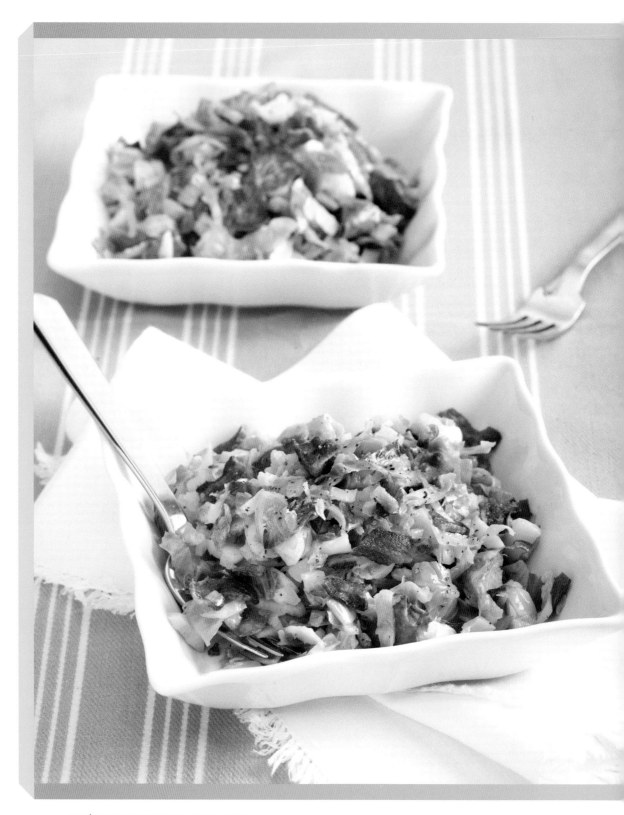

Brussels Sprouts with Crispy Bacon and Shallots

2   center-cut bacon slices, diced
⅓   cup finely chopped shallots (1 large shallot)
1   tablespoon butter
1   pound Brussels sprouts, trimmed, halved, and thinly sliced (5 cups)
¼   cup fat-free, lower-sodium chicken broth
1   tablespoon red wine vinegar
½   teaspoon freshly ground black pepper

1. Cook bacon in a large nonstick skillet over medium heat 3 minutes, stirring often.

2. Using a slotted spoon, remove bacon, reserving drippings in pan; drain bacon. Add shallots to drippings in pan; sauté 1 to 2 minutes or until lightly browned. Add butter and Brussels sprouts; sauté 3 minutes. Add broth; sauté 2 minutes. Stir in vinegar. Remove pan from heat; stir in pepper, and sprinkle with bacon.

YIELD | SERVES 7 (SERVING SIZE: ½ CUP)

CALORIES 70; FAT 4.2g (sat 2.1g, mono 1.3g, poly 0.4g); PROTEIN 3g; CARB 7g; FIBER 2g; CHOL 8mg; IRON 1mg; SODIUM 85mg; CALC 28mg

Roasted Broccoli with Garlic and Anchovy

Minced anchovy fillets deliver bold flavor to this broccoli dish, lending it depth and power.

6	cups broccoli florets (about 1 bunch)
2	tablespoons extra-virgin olive oil, divided
3	garlic cloves, minced
1½	tablespoons butter, melted
2	teaspoons chopped fresh thyme
2	teaspoons grated lemon rind
¾	teaspoon crushed red pepper
2	anchovy fillets, drained and minced
¼	teaspoon kosher salt

1. Preheat oven to 450°.

2. Combine broccoli and 1 tablespoon oil in a large bowl; toss to coat. Place broccoli on a foil-lined baking sheet. Bake at 450° for 6 minutes. Remove from oven; toss with garlic. Bake at 450° for an additional 6 minutes.

3. Place remaining 1 tablespoon oil, butter, and next 4 ingredients (through anchovy) in a large bowl; stir to combine. Add broccoli mixture; toss well to coat. Sprinkle with salt.

YIELD | SERVES 6 (SERVING SIZE: ABOUT ⅔ CUP)

CALORIES 83; FAT 6.9g (sat 1.9g, mono 3.9g, poly 0.7g); PROTEIN 3g; CARB 5g; FIBER 2g; CHOL 6mg; IRON 1mg; SODIUM 165mg; CALCIUM 43mg

Pan-Roasted Asparagus with Lemon Rind

Add a few fresh sage leaves along with the garlic, rosemary, and lemon zest for more herbal flavor. You can serve this at room temperature or chilled. Haricots verts (delicate, thin green beans) work well as a substitute for asparagus.

- 1   **pound asparagus**
- 1   **teaspoon olive oil**
- **Cooking spray**
- 2   **(2-inch) lemon rind strips**
- 2   **garlic cloves, chopped**
- 1   **(1-inch) rosemary sprig**
- ½   **cup water**
- ½   **teaspoon salt**
- ¼   **teaspoon freshly ground black pepper**

1. Snap off tough ends of asparagus.
2. Heat olive oil in a large nonstick skillet coated with cooking spray over medium-high heat. Add asparagus, rind, garlic, and rosemary; sauté 3 minutes or until asparagus is lightly browned.
3. Add ½ cup water to pan; cook 5 minutes or until asparagus is crisp-tender and liquid almost evaporates. Discard rind and rosemary. Sprinkle asparagus with salt and pepper; toss well.

YIELD | SERVES 6 (SERVING SIZE: ABOUT 6 SPEARS)

CALORIES 30; FAT 0.8g (sat 0.1g, mono 0.6g, poly 0.1g); PROTEIN 2g; CARB 4g; FIBER 2g; CHOL 0mg; IRON 0mg; SODIUM 197mg; CALCIUM 20mg

Spring Vegetable Skillet

A hot skillet allows you to control the degree of doneness more precisely, and the intense heat helps seal in flavor.

16   **baby carrots with tops (about 10 ounces)**
¾   **teaspoon kosher salt, divided**
12   **ounces sugar snap peas, trimmed**
1½   **tablespoons olive oil**
1   **tablespoon chopped fresh tarragon**
¼   **teaspoon freshly ground black pepper**
1   **teaspoon grated lemon rind**
1   **teaspoon fresh lemon juice**

1. Peel carrots, and cut off tops to within 1 inch of carrot; cut in half lengthwise.

2. Place ¼ teaspoon salt in a large saucepan of water; bring to a boil. Add carrots and peas; cook 3 minutes or until crisp-tender. Drain.

3. Heat oil in a large nonstick skillet over medium-high heat. Add vegetables, and cook 1 minute, stirring to coat. Stir in remaining ½ teaspoon salt, tarragon, and pepper; cook 1 minute. Remove from heat; stir in rind and juice.

YIELD | SERVES 6 (SERVING SIZE: ²/₃ CUP)

CALORIES 69; FAT 2.9g (sat 1.8g mono 0.7g, poly 0.1g); PROTEIN 2g; CARB 9g; FIBER 3g; CHOL 8mg; IRON 1mg; SODIUM 221mg; CALCIUM 58mg

Grilled Vegetable Antipasto

Grilling the zucchini and eggplant makes them more absorbent, which allows them to soak up more of the flavorful vinaigrette.

2	red bell peppers
2	zucchini, each cut in half lengthwise (about 1 pound)
2	Japanese eggplant, each cut in half lengthwise (about 8 ounces)
¼	cup chopped fresh parsley
¼	cup balsamic vinegar
1	tablespoon extra-virgin olive oil
¼	teaspoon salt
6	garlic cloves, peeled and crushed

1. Prepare grill.
2. Place peppers on grill rack; grill 15 minutes or until charred, turning occasionally. Place peppers in a zip-top plastic bag; seal and let stand 15 minutes. Peel peppers; discard seeds and membranes. Coarsely chop peppers; place in a large zip-top plastic bag. Place zucchini and eggplant on grill rack; grill 10 minutes, turning occasionally. Remove zucchini and eggplant from grill; let stand 10 minutes. Coarsely chop zucchini and eggplant; add to chopped peppers.
3. Combine parsley and remaining ingredients, stirring with a whisk. Pour the parsley mixture over pepper mixture. Seal bag; toss gently to coat. Refrigerate at least 2 hours or overnight.

YIELD | SERVES 4 (SERVING SIZE: 1 CUP)

CALORIES 122; FAT 4g (sat 0.6g, mono 2.5g, poly 0.6g); PROTEIN 4g; CARB 21g; FIBER 7g; CHOL 0mg; IRON 2mg; SODIUM 163mg; CALCIUM 52mg

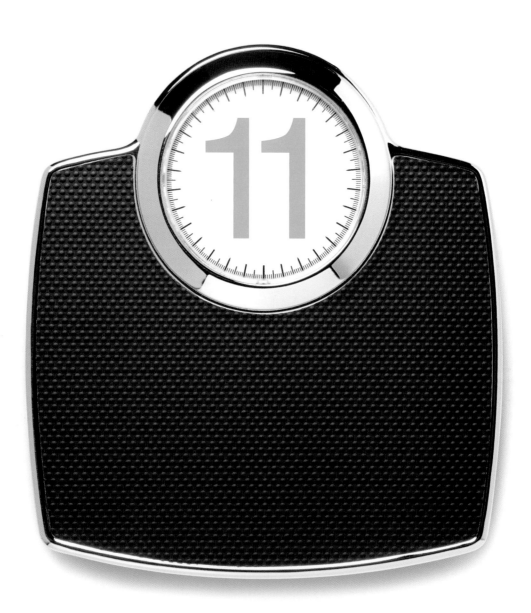

JUST BECAUSE YOU'VE GONE PALEO doesn't mean you have to forgo the occasional sweet treat or cocktail. Make room for a few indulgences here and there to help you never feel deprived. Here are some refreshing frozen desserts, decadent baked goods, and boozy beverages that won't sabotage your weight-loss efforts, if enjoyed in moderation.

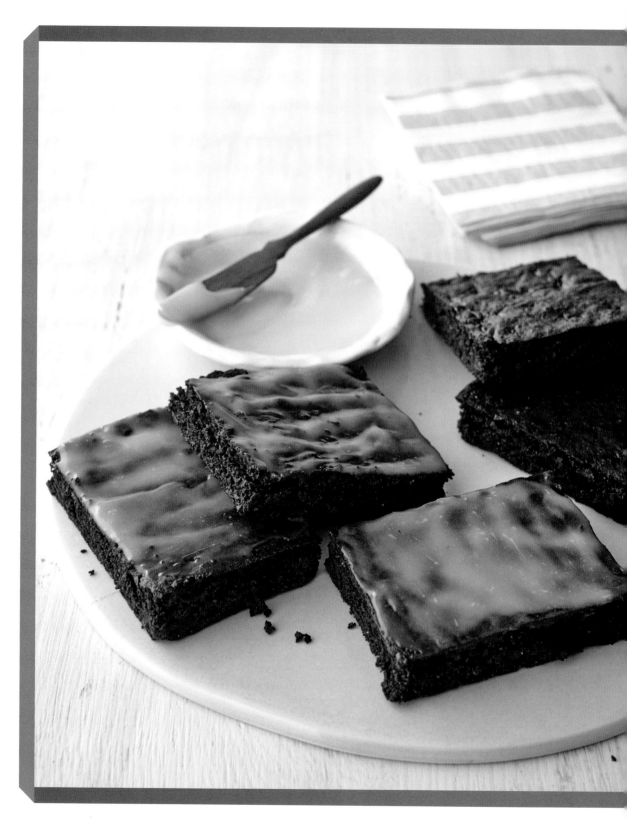

Brownies

The dates are the secret to these rich brownies' ooey-gooey texture.

1	cup walnuts
½	cup unsweetened cocoa powder
¼	cup organic coconut powder
1	tablespoon cinnamon
½	teaspoon baking soda
½	teaspoon salt
½	cup Medjool dates, pitted
½	cup honey
3	large eggs, lightly beaten
	Coconut oil
1	cup coconut cream concentrate (melted)

1. Preheat oven to 325°.
2. Place walnuts and next 5 ingredients (through salt) in a food processor; pulse until ground. Add dates and honey; pulse until smooth.
3. Combine walnut mixture and eggs in a bowl; stir until mixed well.
4. Pour into a 9 x 13-inch baking dish greased with coconut oil. Bake at 325° for 25 to 30 minutes or until a wooden toothpick inserted in center comes out clean without moist crumbs clinging.
5. Cool pan on rack. Spread coconut cream concentrate over brownies. Cut into squares.

YIELD | SERVES 8 (SERVING SIZE: 1 SQUARE)

CALORIES 362; FAT 19g (sat 7g, mono 2g, poly 7.3g); PROTEIN 7g; CARB 39g; FIBER 4g; CHOL 70mg; IRON 1mg; SODIUM 131mg; CALC 39mg

SIMPLE SWAPS
Have Your Cake

Thanks to hard work by Paleo enthusiasts, you can find recipes for cakes, cookies, and even banana bread without too much trouble. Almond flour, coconut oil, maple syrup, and honey will be the trick to producing baked goods anyone—Paleo or not—can love.

Lemon Squares

Tender, short cookie crust meets a luscious, tart, lemony topping in these decadent treats.

Crust:
- 4 cups almond flour
- ½ cup arrowroot starch
- ½ teaspoon salt
- ½ teaspoon baking soda
- ½ cup pure maple syrup or honey
- 2 teaspoons pure vanilla extract
- 1 cup coconut oil, melted

Topping:
- 4 eggs
- ¾ cup pure maple syrup or honey
- ½ cup fresh lemon juice
- 1 tablespoon lemon zest
- 1 tablespoon arrowroot starch

1. Preheat oven to 325°.

2. To prepare crust, combine almond flour and next 6 ingredients (through coconut oil). Press mixture into a 9 x 13-inch pan greased with coconut oil. Bake at 325° for 20 minutes or until golden brown.

3. While crust is baking, prepare topping. Combine eggs and next 4 ingredients (through arrowroot starch) in a large bowl, stirring with a whisk until smooth. Pour lemon mixture over baked crust. Bake 20 minutes or until set. Cool on rack. Cover and chill 2 hours.

YIELD | SERVES 16 (SERVING SIZE: 1 SQUARE)

CALORIES 378; FAT 29g (sat 13g, mono 7.8g, poly 6g); PROTEIN 8g; CARB 27g; FIBER 3g; CHOL 47mg; IRON 1mg; SODIUM 134mg; CALC 94mg

SIMPLE SWAPS

Crust Concern?

When making pies or tarts, you can get creative with the crust by using coconut or almond flour; crushed almonds, pecans, or walnuts; and lard. You won't miss the traditional white flour crust, and you may be able to get away without baking, depending on the filling.

Coconut Custard

This creamy coconut custard should be made the night before. Sprinkle with cinnamon before serving. We strained the custard before chilling to ensure it would be smooth.

- ¾ cup honey
- ½ cup arrowroot starch
- ⅛ teaspoon salt
- 3 (13.5-ounce) cans light coconut milk
- ½ teaspoon vanilla extract
- ⅛ teaspoon coconut extract
- ⅛ teaspoon ground cinnamon

1. Combine first 4 ingredients in a heavy medium saucepan. Bring to a boil over medium heat; cook for 1 minute, stirring constantly. Remove from heat; stir in extracts. Strain through a sieve into a shallow 2-quart dish; cover surface of custard with plastic wrap. Chill overnight. Sprinkle with cinnamon before serving.

YIELD | SERVES 10 (SERVING SIZE: ABOUT ⅔ CUP)

CALORIES 174; FAT 6g (sat 4.5g, mono 0.5g, poly 0.5g); PROTEIN 0g; CARB 32g; FIBER 1g; CHOL 0mg; IRON 0mg; SODIUM 68mg; CALC 2mg

SIMPLE SWAPS
Cool Custard

Coconut milk can stand in for dairy in sweet sauces and custards. Otherwise, the eggs, vanilla, and any fruit you might add will, of course, be fine, and you can use honey instead of refined sugar.

Avocado Lime Cheesecake

⅓ cup almonds
¼ cup shredded unsweetened coconut
2 dates, pitted
1 teaspoon water
1 teaspoon melted coconut oil
2 large avocados
6 tablespoons coconut nectar
½ cup fresh lime juice
1 tablespoon honey
5 tablespoons melted coconut oil
4 tablespoons melted coconut butter
¼ teaspoon lime zest

1. Place almonds in food processor; pulse until almonds are ground. Add coconut, dates, and 1 teaspoon water; pulse until dough forms. Add coconut oil; pulse until oil is incorporated into dough.

2. Press dough into the bottom of a 6-inch springform pan; set aside.

3. Combine avocados, nectar, juice, and honey until smooth and creamy. Add oil, butter, and zest. Blend to incorporate. Pour over crust. Chill 8 hours.

YIELD | SERVES 12 (SERVING SIZE: 1 SLICE)

CALORIES 208; FAT 19.4g (sat 14.4g, mono 2.4g, poly 1g); PROTEIN 2g; CARB 10g; FIBER 3g; CHOL 3mg; IRON 1mg; SODIUM 4mg; CALC 19mg

Avocado Ice Pops

They're a fruit and creamy-rich—perfect for freezing on a stick.

- ¼ **cup water**
- 6 **tablespoons honey**
- 2 **cups chopped, peeled avocado**
- ½ **teaspoon grated lime rind**
- 2 **tablespoons lime juice**
- ⅛ **teaspoon kosher salt**

1. Combine ¼ cup water and honey in a saucepan over medium heat. Cook 4 minutes, stirring to dissolve agave. Remove from heat; cool to room temperature. Place honey mixture, avocado, rind, juice, and salt in a food processor; process until smooth. Divide mixture evenly among 6 (4-ounce) ice-pop molds. Top with lid. Freeze 4 hours or until thoroughly frozen.

YIELD | SERVES 6 (SERVING SIZE: 1 ICE POP)

CALORIES 130; FAT 7.3g (sat 1.1g, mono 4.9g, poly 1g); PROTEIN 1g; CARB 17g; FIBER 3g; CHOL 0mg; IRON 0mg; SODIUM 44mg; CALC 7mg

SIMPLE SWAPS

Avocado for dessert?

It really works, believe it or not. When you need to give a dessert richness and creaminess, avocados can serve the purpose. Cheesecake knockoff? Mash in some avocados. Mousse? Again, that smooth avocado texture can help you achieve the result you need.

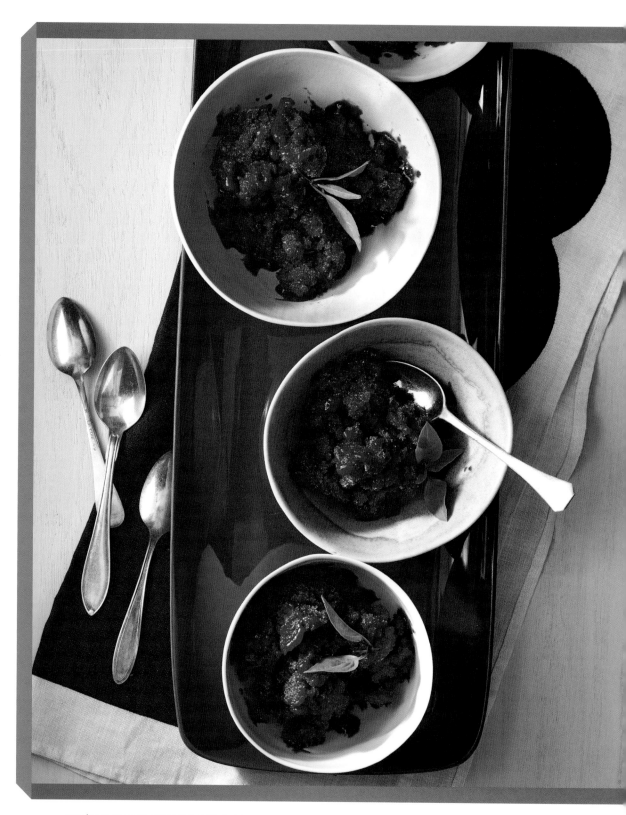

Basil Plum Granita

Although complex black plums, with their winey flavor, taste and look spectacular in this refreshing granita, you can use most any variety.

1	cup water
⅔	cup honey
¼	teaspoon vanilla extract
⅛	teaspoon salt
5	whole allspice
1½	pounds black plums, quartered and pitted
2	tablespoons fresh lime juice
¾	cup basil leaves

1. Place first 6 ingredients in a large saucepan over medium-high heat; bring to a boil. Reduce heat; simmer for 15 minutes or until plums begin to fall apart, stirring occasionally. Place pan in a large ice-filled bowl; cool completely, stirring occasionally. Discard allspice.

2. Place the plum mixture, lime juice, and basil in a blender; process until well blended. Press the plum mixture through a fine sieve over a bowl, and discard solids. Pour the mixture into an 8-inch square glass or ceramic baking dish. Cover and freeze until partially frozen (about 2 hours). Scrape with a fork, crushing any lumps. Freeze for 3 hours, scraping with a fork every hour, or until completely frozen.

YIELD | SERVES 8 (SERVING SIZE: ABOUT ½ CUP)

CALORIES 107; FAT 0g (sat 0g, mono 0g, poly 0g); PROTEIN 0g; CARB 23g; FIBER 1g; CHOL 0mg; IRON 0mg; SODIUM 38mg; CALC 9mg

Spicy Mango Granita

Finish off the evening with a spicy-sweet iced dessert featuring mango, orange juice, and fresh lime juice. Garnish with additional red pepper for more kick.

4	cups cubed, peeled ripe mango
6	tablespoons honey
¼	cup fresh orange juice
3	tablespoons fresh lime juice
⅜	teaspoon ground red pepper
Dash of salt	

1. Combine all ingredients in a small saucepan; bring to a boil. Reduce heat, and simmer 10 minutes. Remove from heat; let stand 10 minutes. Pour mixture into a blender; process until smooth. Strain through a sieve over a bowl, and discard solids. Pour into an 11 x 7-inch baking dish; cool. Cover and freeze for 45 minutes; scrape with a fork. Freeze. Scrape every 45 minutes until completely frozen (about 6 hours). Remove from freezer; scrape with a fork until fluffy.

YIELD | SERVES 6 (SERVING SIZE: ABOUT ½ CUP)

CALORIES 136; FAT 0g (sat 0g, mono 0g, poly 0g); PROTEIN 1g; CARB 35g; FIBER 2g; CHOL 0mg; IRON 0mg; SODIUM 2mg; CALC 15mg

Island Sunrise Smoothie

Play with your food: Have fun by serving smaller portions in hollowed-out limes.

2	cups chopped papaya
½	cup orange juice
1	tablespoon honey
2	teaspoons fresh lime juice
Pinch of salt	
1	cup frozen (½-inch) cubed mango
1	cup frozen strawberries

1. Place first 5 ingredients in a blender; process until smooth. Add mango and strawberries; process until smooth.

YIELD | SERVES 3 (SERVING SIZE: 1 CUP)

CALORIES 131; FAT 0.7g (sat 0.2g, mono 0.2g, poly 0.2g); PROTEIN 2g; CARB 33g; FIBER 4g; CHOL 0mg; IRON 1mg; SODIUM 59mg; CALC 39mg

Triple Melon Smoothie

Melons are at their peak season June through September. Make this smoothie with ripe, in-season fruit for a great-tasting, refreshing drink when the weather's hot. Garnish with additional diced melon, if desired.

2½ cups chopped, seedless watermelon
½   cup fresh orange juice
2   teaspoon honey
2½ cups (1-inch) cubed cantaloupe, frozen
1   cup (1-inch) cubed honeydew melon, frozen

1. Place first 3 ingredients in a blender; process until smooth.
2. Remove center piece of blender lid; secure blender lid on blender. With blender on, drop cantaloupe and honeydew through the center of lid; process until smooth.

YIELD | SERVES 4 (SERVING SIZE: 1 CUP)

CALORIES 102; FAT 0.5g (sat 0.1g, mono 0.1g, poly 0.2g); PROTEIN 2g; CARB 25g; FIBER 2g; CHOL 0mg; IRON 1mg; SODIUM 25mg; CALC 22mg

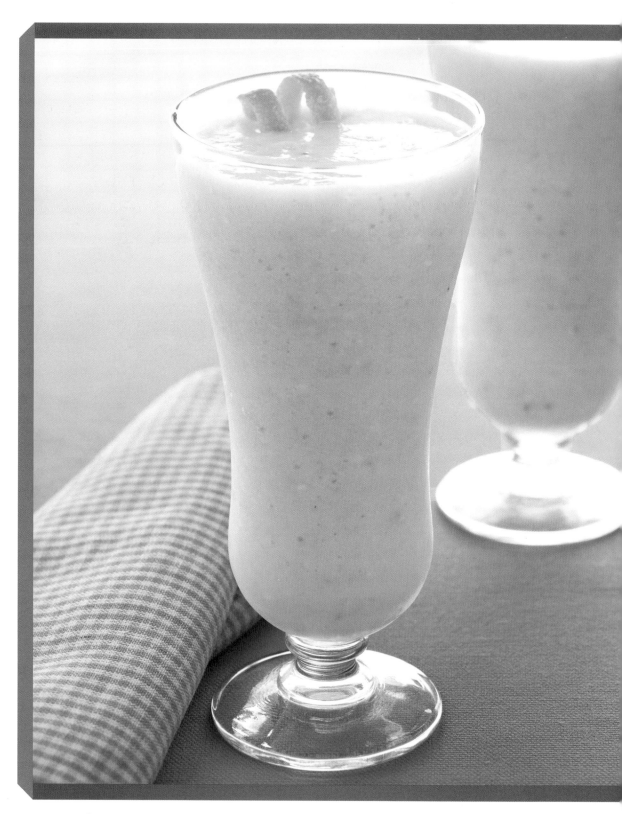

Orange, Banana, and Pineapple Frappé

A frappé is similar to a fruit juice or other liquid smoothie, but it's made with a larger proportion of fruit than dairy. Garnish with a twist of orange zest, if desired. To skip the dairy, substitute unsweetened vanilla cultured coconut milk for the low-fat yogurt.

2⅔ cups frozen sliced bananas (about 3 medium bananas)
¾   cup pineapple juice
½   cup orange sections (about 1 large orange)
½   cup coconut milk
1   tablespoon flaked sweetened coconut
2   tablespoons fresh orange juice
1   cup fresh pineapple chunks

1. Place all ingredients in a blender; process until smooth. Serve immediately.

YIELD | SERVES 4 (SERVING SIZE: ABOUT 1 CUP)

CALORIES 194; FAT 1.3g (sat 0.8g, mono 0.2g, poly 0.1g); PROTEIN 4g; CARB 46g; FIBER 4g; CHOL 2mg; IRON 1mg; SODIUM 28mg; CALC 90mg

Gingered Tropical Fruit Salad

Section the oranges over a bowl, and reserve the juice to make this dressing for the salad.

2	tablespoons fresh orange juice
2	tablespoons fresh lime juice
1	tablespoon honey
1	teaspoon grated peeled fresh ginger
2	cups cubed fresh pineapple
¾	cup sliced peeled kiwifruit (about 2 kiwifruit)
1	large navel orange, peeled and sectioned
¼	cup flaked unsweetened coconut, toasted

1. Combine first 4 ingredients in a large bowl. Add pineapple, kiwifruit, and orange; toss gently to coat. Sprinkle with coconut. Cover and chill until ready to serve.

YIELD | SERVES 6 (SERVING SIZE: ABOUT ½ CUP)

CALORIES 85; FAT 1.3g (sat 0.9g, mono 0.1g, poly 0g); PROTEIN 1g; CARB 19g; FIBER 2g; CHOL 0mg; IRON 0mg; SODIUM 11mg; CALC 26mg

Roasted Nectarines with Coconut Custard

Roasting the nectarines concentrates their natural sugar, and they're especially fine served with this egg-rich sauce. Peaches or plums also roast well.

Sauce:
⅛   **teaspoon salt**
4   **egg yolks**
⅓   **cup honey**
1   **cup plus 2 tablespoons coconut milk**
¼   **teaspoon vanilla extract**
Nectarines:
6   **medium nectarines, halved and pitted (about 2 pounds)**
Cooking spray
1   **tablespoon honey**
Verbena sprigs (optional)

1. To prepare sauce, combine salt and egg yolks in a medium bowl. Gradually add ⅓ cup honey, beating 2 minutes with a mixer at medium-high speed.

2. Heat 1 cup coconut milk over medium heat in a small, heavy saucepan to 180° or until tiny bubbles form around edge (do not boil). Gradually add hot milk to honey mixture, stirring constantly. Return milk mixture to pan; cook over medium-low heat 5 minutes or until slightly thick and mixture coats the back of a spoon, stirring constantly (do not boil). Remove from heat. Stir in remaining 2 tablespoons coconut milk and vanilla. Place pan in a large ice-filled bowl until mixture cools completely, stirring occasionally. Spoon mixture into a bowl. Cover and chill.

3. Preheat oven to 400°.

4. To prepare nectarines, place nectarines, cut sides up, in a 9 x 13-inch baking dish coated with cooking spray. Drizzle nectarines evenly with 1 tablespoon honey. Bake at 400° for 25 minutes or until nectarines are soft and lightly browned. Serve with chilled sauce. Garnish with verbena sprigs, if desired.

YIELD | SERVES 6 (SERVING SIZE 2 NECTARINE HALVES AND ¼ CUP SAUCE)

CALORIES 279; FAT 6.7g (sat 3g, mono 2g, poly 1.5g); PROTEIN 5.3g; CARB 55g; FIBER 4g; CHOL 125mg; IRON 1mg; SODIUM 87mg; CALC 66mg

Cider Sangria

It's fine to make this punch ahead; just hold off on adding the apple cider—which adds bright and effervescent notes—until right before serving.

½	cup water
¼	cup honey
3	cinnamon sticks
¾	cup brandy
1	apple, cored and diced
1	pear, cored and diced
1	cup black seedless or Concord grapes
3½	cups leftover dry white wine, such as sauvignon blanc (a little more than 1 [750-milliliter] bottle)
1¾	cups certified organic sparkling apple-cranberry cider (such as Martinelli's)

1. Combine ½ cup water, honey, and cinnamon sticks in a small saucepan over medium-high heat; cook until honey dissolves, stirring as needed. Pour mixture into a large bowl; cool for about 10 minutes. Stir in brandy. Add diced apple and pear; toss to coat. Cool completely.
2. Strain brandy mixture into a large pitcher, reserving apples and pears. Discard cinnamon sticks. Thread apples, pears, and grapes onto 10 short skewers or cocktail picks. Return any remaining fruit to the pitcher. Stir in wine and cider. Fill 10 glasses with ice. Divide punch evenly among glasses; garnish each glass with a fruit skewer.

YIELD | SERVES 10 (SERVING SIZE: ABOUT ¾ CUP)

CALORIES 175; FAT 0g (sat 0g, mono 0g, poly 0g); PROTEIN 0g; CARB 22g; FIBER 2g; CHOL 0mg; IRON 4mg; SODIUM 5mg; CALC 13mg

Mulled Wine Sangria

You'll love the heady flavors in this version of the classic Spanish drink. It's a good make-ahead option for entertaining; add the club soda just before serving.

2	teaspoons whole allspice
¼	teaspoon whole cloves
1	(3-inch) cinnamon stick, broken in half
1	(3 x 1-inch) strip orange rind
1	(750-milliliter) bottle merlot or other red wine, chilled and divided
⅓	cup honey
1	sachet Mulling Spice Blend
½	cup fresh orange juice (about 1 large orange)
1	(16-ounce) bag frozen unsweetened strawberries
½	orange, thinly sliced and cut in half
1	(12-ounce) can club soda

1. Combine whole allspice and next 3 ingredients (through orange rind) on a double layer of cheesecloth. Gather edges of cheesecloth together; tie securely.

2. Combine 1 cup wine, honey, and sachet in a small saucepan; bring to a simmer. Cook 5 minutes. Remove from heat; cool. Discard sachet. Pour mixture into a pitcher; add remaining 3 cups wine. Chill thoroughly. Add juice, strawberries, orange slices, and club soda.

YIELD | SERVES 8 (SERVING SIZE: 1 CUP)

CALORIES 143; FAT 0g (sat 0g, mono 0g, poly 0g); PROTEIN 0g; CARB 19g; FIBER 1g; CHOL 0mg; IRON 1mg; SODIUM 14mg; CALC 24mg

SIMPLE SWAPS
Avoid sweet wines

Choose the drier varietals such as cabernet sauvignon, Côtes du Rhône, and pinot noir for reds; for whites, stick to pinot gris, pinot grigio, or sauvignon blanc.

Sparkling Rosemary-Peach Cocktails

A heady punch of woodsy rosemary creates an herbaceous riff on the classic Bellini.

¾	**cup water**
½	**cup agave nectar or honey**
1	**(3-inch) rosemary sprig**
2	**ripe peeled peaches, cut into 1-inch pieces**
1	**(750-milliliter) bottle Champagne or sparkling wine, chilled**

1. Combine first 3 ingredients in a small saucepan; bring to a boil. Remove from heat; cool to room temperature. Strain rosemary syrup in a sieve over a bowl; discard solids. Cover and chill at least 1 hour.

2. Place rosemary syrup and peaches in a blender, and process until smooth. Strain mixture through a sieve over a bowl; cover and chill at least 4 hours. Spoon about 2 tablespoons peach syrup into each of 8 Champagne flutes, and top each serving with about ⅓ cup Champagne.

YIELD | SERVES 8 (SERVING SIZE: 1 CUP)

CALORIES 126; FAT 0g (sat 0g, mono 0g, poly 0g); PROTEIN 0g; CARB 17g; FIBER 0g; CHOL 0mg; IRON 0mg; SODIUM 1mg; CALC 3mg

Cucumber-Mint Tequila Tonic

This is the perfect warm-weather cocktail. Made with fresh mint, cilantro leaves, and chopped cucumber, it's refreshing and fabulous.

- 2   cups chopped English cucumber
- ½   cup mint leaves
- ⅓   cup agave nectar
- ¼   cup cilantro leaves
- 1   lime, sectioned and juiced
- Dash of salt
- ½   cup tequila blanco
- ¾   cup chilled tonic water

1. Combine first 6 ingredients in a food processor; pulse until smooth. Scrape mixture into a bowl; stir in tequila. Chill. Strain. Stir in tonic water. Serve over ice.

YIELD | SERVES 6 (SERVING SIZE: ABOUT ⅓ CUP)

CALORIES 114; FAT 0g (sat 0g, mono 0g, poly 0g); PROTEIN 0g; CARB 19g; FIBER 1g; CHOL 0mg; IRON 0mg; SODIUM 45mg; CALC 0mg

SIMPLE SWAPS
Know Your Spirits

Going cold turkey will be tough for oenophiles and others who cherish an evening drink. While cutting out alcohol is a good idea for your liver and your Paleo diet, if you feel the need to imbibe and you aren't a big fan of hard cider, look for alcohols that aren't grain-based. These include vodka, red wine, white wine, rum, and tequila.

PART 3

LIVING THE PALEO LIFESTYLE

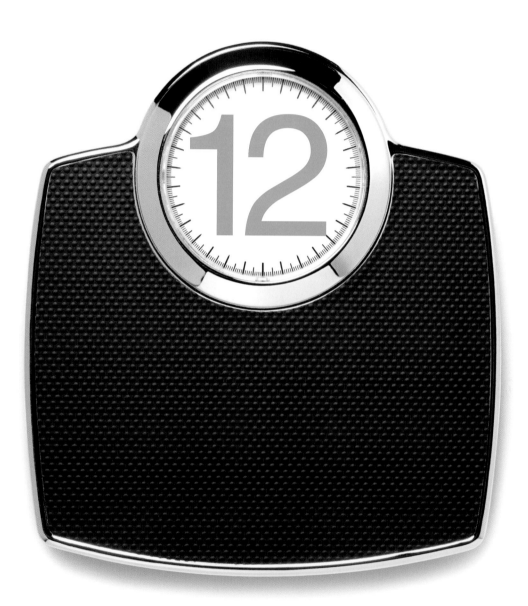

TO FULLY EMBRACE THE Paleo way, the next step is Paleo exercise. As you shift your diet to this high-energy, high-protein approach, your body will crave and respond to a Paleo routine that helps you get—and stay—fit. You'll be happy to learn that you won't have to trudge on a treadmill for hours or start scheduling marathons.

Our Paleo ancestors would have been truly puzzled by our modern approach to exercise only because they didn't have to schedule or plan their activity: It was an integral part of everyday life. They had to chase down prey, haul water, build shelter, and forage for fruit and vegetables. Their survival required a full day's worth of cross training, almost every day.

Pairing the high-protein, pure-energy Paleo eating plan with the Paleo fitness approach will do wonders for your body and your weight loss. The first step is to start building more activity into your typical day. For example, if you work in an office, try out a standing desk. Or, if that's not possible, look for opportunities to stand and move whenever possible. This could mean taking calls while standing or answering interoffice messages in person. Instead of tapping out an email or instant message, get up and walk over to your correspondent. You'll not only get more activity, but your officemates will also probably appreciate the face-to-face contact.

As for actual exercise, the goal with the Paleo approach is to find active ways to play so that your workouts never feel like an obligation. The problem with our modern-day exercise is that it's usually one more chore out of many, and we happily put it off when something—anything—better presents itself. For that reason, you'll want to find activities that you love so much that you can't bear not doing them.

The reason playing games—or just playing—works so well for Paleo exercise is that it usually involves quick bursts and brief rests. Think about most of the physical games we play: tennis, racquetball, basketball, soccer—they all require quick, explosive efforts broken up by brief rests. The great thing about this approach to exercise is that you can include tag and wrestling with the kids or a pet. The ideal exercise involves brief, intense bursts, like running after a ball or pursuing someone, that are broken up with pauses in the action that allow you to catch your breath, such as when you're between points or rallies or while you're lying on the grass laughing.

Why is this start-stop approach important? Mostly because it nicely mimics Paleo activity, the kind of effort that best suits our bodies from an evolutionary perspective. But even better, researchers have found that breaking up your activity like this leads to more weight loss and improved fitness. Exercise scientists refer to this type of exercise as HIIT: high-intensity interval training. In study after study researchers have found it far outperforms standard, steady-paced cardio. Another plus is that exercising this way is more fun.

In a 2011 study published in the *Journal of Obesity,* researchers reviewed all the research available on HIIT and found that it trumped steady-paced exercise in every possible measure. Interval training increased fitness and fat-burning capacity more than regular exercise, and it accomplished these results in about half the time. (A typical interval-based workout runs 20 to 30 minutes, while steady-paced sessions usually run 40 to 60 minutes.) Even better for dieters, one study indicated that interval training led to at least three times the weight loss of steady-paced aerobics. Interval training also seems to target abdominal fat—your belly—which envelops organs and can lead to chronic disease and subcutaneous fat.

There are more benefits to interval training: According to the American College of Sports Medicine, you can elevate your metabolism for up to 24 hours post-exercise by doing intervals. By injecting brief periods of intense effort into your exercise (either by playing fast-paced games or adding some jogging and sprinting into your regular walks, runs, swims, or cycling), you can kick your metabolism up a notch during your workout—and it takes hours for it to slow down again. That equals ongoing calorie burn long after you've showered and toweled off.

Beef Up Your Exercise

The other important aspect of Paleo and overall health is to be strong. All activity prescriptions, whether they come from Paleo proponents or general health experts, include strength training. But again, what sets Paleo apart is the approach to building muscle.

Instead of doing three sets of light lifts and spending hours and days in the gym, Paleo again lends itself to briefer, more intense weight lifting. You don't even need equipment; you could use the resistance provided by your own body weight to create a complete full-body regimen. Pushups, pullups, crunches, lunges, squats, and calf raises, and you're done.

However, many people find going to a gym can help you stay committed to a program. Check out BodyPump or cardio-strength classes to simulate a Paleo strength regimen, or explore more old-school techniques like using kettlebells or CrossFit (which is hugely popular among Paleo dieters).

Strength training will also help you shed pounds faster while making your body look better. In 2010, Australian researchers reported that when overweight dieters added strength training three times a week, they lost much more weight than people who only dieted. After four months, the strength-training group had dropped an average of 30 pounds—10 pounds more than those who only dieted. What's more, the lifters shaved 5.5 inches off their waistlines, compared to just 3.5 inches in the diet-only group. The exercises included just eight moves: shoulder, chest, tricep, and leg presses, seated rows, knee extensions, lat pulldowns, and situps. You can do most of these lifts (or variations of them) at home with a pair of dumbbells. Or you can substitute other strength-building workouts.

Adding Intervals to Your Exercise

Obviously, the best way to build in interval training is to pick up a sport that naturally requires brief bursts of intense effort. But you can't play tennis or basketball all the time. You may not even enjoy those kinds of endeavors.

But you can still make intervals part of your workout by mixing them into your usual pursuit. If you're a walker and you typically exercise for 30 minutes, every 5 minutes try adding a burst of jogging or fast walking for 30 seconds. As you become more fit, you can increase the interval length to a minute and decrease the walking segments to 2 minutes. For the biggest metabolism boost, you'll want to make sure that the interval portion leaves you breathing hard. (By the way, if you haven't been exercising regularly and have any risk factors for heart disease, such as obesity or high blood pressure, check with your doctor before you start an interval program.)

You can set a goal of working toward a more challenging interval sequence, such as "10-20-30" (or, more accurately, "30-20-10"). The concept is that after a proper warmup, you do 30 seconds of your activity—walking, jogging, swimming, and so forth—at a light, easy-to-maintain pace. Then do 20 seconds of normal-level intensity, and end the minute with 10 seconds of all-out effort before going back to 30 seconds of light effort. The advantage of this approach is that after 5 to 10 minutes, you'll get a very thorough and demanding workout. You can go longer of course, but just 10 minutes of this leads to improved stamina, according to the Danish researchers at the University of Copenhagen who developed this approach.

For the strength-building exercise portion of your workouts, consider lifting heavier weights than most people typically do (or want to). How much weight is enough? In the program below, you'll do two sets of each move. You should choose a weight heavy enough so that your muscles are spent after the second set.

Complete two sets of 8 to 12 repetitions with a 1-minute rest between sets. Schedule workouts at least twice a week, but make sure you have a day off between sessions to give your muscles a chance to recover.

1. Chest press
2. Squats
3. Shoulder press
4. Crunches
5. Calf raises
6. Dumbbell squats
7. Biceps curls
8. Triceps kickbacks
9. Bent-over rows
10. Dumbbell lunge

Chest press

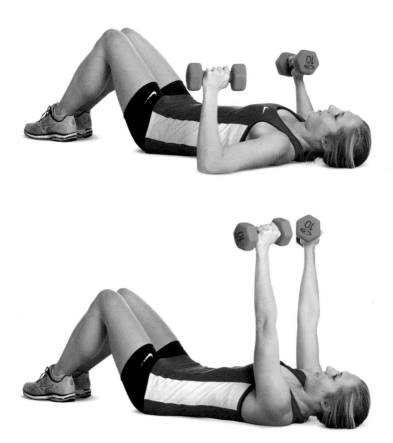

1. Lie on the floor face up with your feet firmly on the ground, your back relaxed. Grasp a pair of dumbbells and with arms bent hold the dumbbells above your chest with your palms facing forward and your thumbs wrapped around each weight.

2. Exhale and slowly press the dumbbells straight up so they are over your shoulders. Wrists should remain in a neutral position (do not bend them throughout the exercise). Be careful not to arch your back. Inhale as you slowly lower the dumbbells back to starting position.

Squats

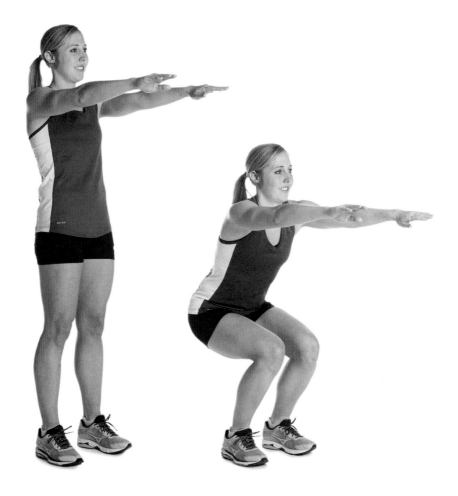

1. Stretch your arms straight out in front of your chest with palms facing the floor. Spread feet until they are hip-width apart.

2. Squat by slowly bending your knees and pushing back hips until your thighs are parallel to the floor. Pause, then slowly return to starting position.

Shoulder press

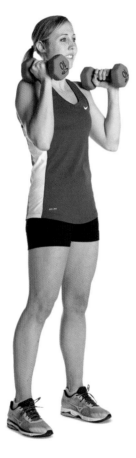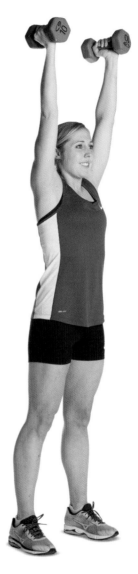

1. Hold a dumbbell in each hand, and stand with your feet hip-width apart. Brace your torso by contracting your abdominal muscles. Exhale and slowly lift the dumbbells until they are level with your shoulders. Palms should be facing in and thumbs should be wrapped around the handles. Wrists should remain in a neutral position (do not bend them throughout the exercise). Pull your shoulder blades down and back.

2. Exhale and press the dumbbells overhead until your elbows are straight, taking care not to arch your back. Inhale and slowly lower the dumbbells to shoulder height.

Crunches

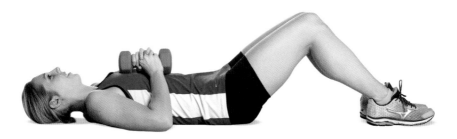

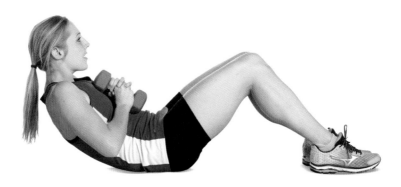

1. Lie face-up on the floor with your knees bent, feet flat on the floor and heels a comfortable distance away from your rear. Grasp a dumbbell vertically against your chest with both hands.

2. Engage your abdominal muscles and exhale as you slowly raise your head and shoulders off the floor and draw your rib cage toward your pelvis. Continue until your mid back is lifted off the floor. Pause at the top of the motion, then slowly lower your head and shoulders back to the mat as you inhale. Repeat for 60 seconds.

Note: This exercise can also be done without weights.

Calf raises

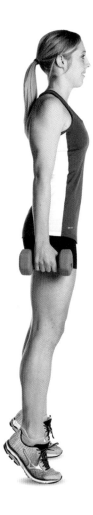

1. Stand holding a dumbbell in each hand. Spread your feet so they are hip-width apart. Keep your back straight and tighten your abs.

2. Exhale and slowly rise onto the balls of your feet, keeping your knees straight but not locked. At the top, pause and squeeze your calves. Inhale and lower yourself to the ground. Repeat step 2.

Note: This exercise can also be done without weights.

Dumbbell squats

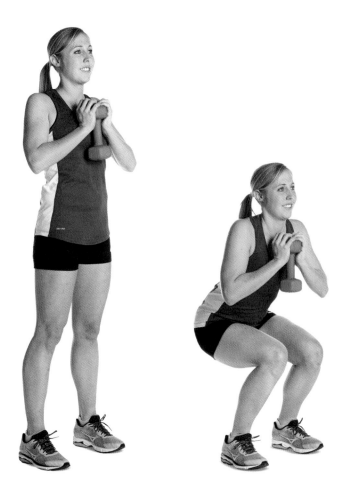

1. Grasp a dumbbell vertically in front of your chest with both hands, and point elbows to the floor. Spread feet until they are hip-width apart.

2. Inhale and squat by slowly pushing back hips and bending your knees. Squat only as low as you feel comfortable or until your thighs are parallel to the floor. Pause, then exhale and slowly return to starting position.

Note: This exercise can also be done without weights.

Biceps curls

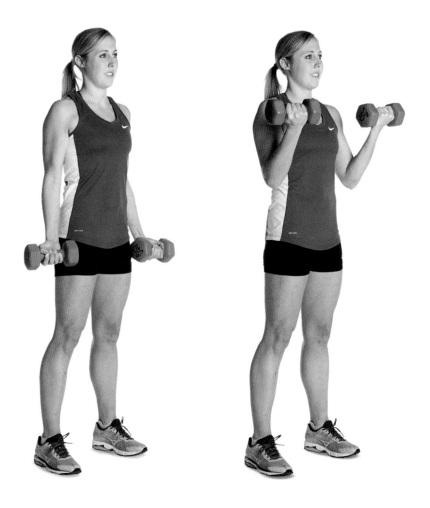

1. Stand with your feet hip-width apart and grasp a pair of dumbbells with palms facing forward and your thumbs wrapped around each weight. Keep your back straight, your abdominals tight, and your shoulders down and back.

2. Bending at your elbows, exhale and pull the dumbbells directly up until they are level with the top of your chest. Pause at the top of the movement. Inhale and slowly lower the dumbbells to the starting position.

Triceps kickbacks

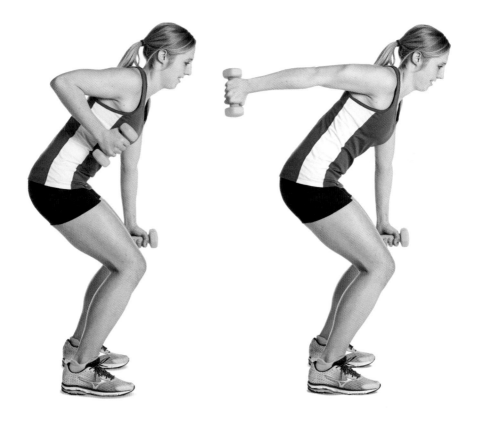

1. Grasp a pair of dumbbells with palms facing each other, thumbs wrapped around each weight. Spread your feet so they are hip-width apart and lean slightly forward, allowing dumbbells to hang.

2. Exhale and bend your right elbow and draw the dumbbell up to your side, making your upper arm parallel with the floor. Extend the dumbbell back to bring your forearm in line with your upper arm. Inhale and reverse the movement slowly by bending your elbow. Do 12 to 15 reps with each arm.

Bent-over rows

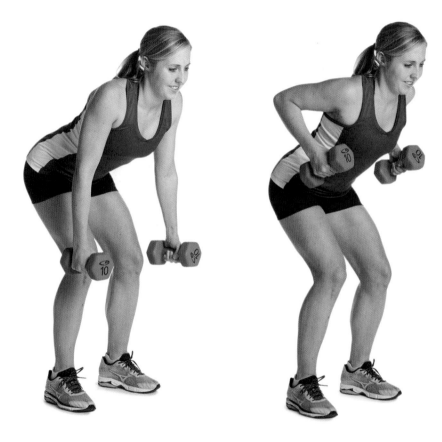

1. Hold a dumbbell in each hand with your palms facing each other. Spread your feet hip-width apart, and slightly bend your knees. Slowly tilt your torso forward, keeping your back straight until your chest is almost parallel to the floor. Allow your arms to hang perpendicular to the floor.

2. Exhale and bend your elbows to pull the dumbbells up, squeezing your shoulder blades together and taking care not to arch your back. Inhale and slowly lower the dumbbells to the starting position.

Dumbbell lunge

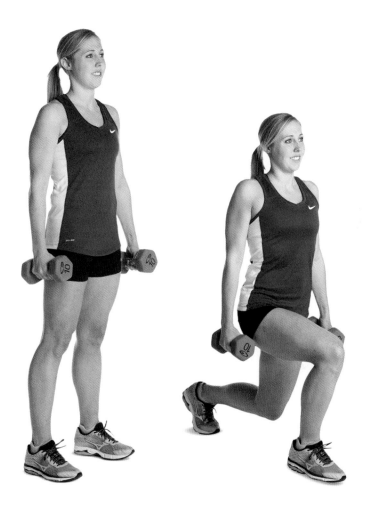

1. Stand with your feet hip-width apart, toes facing forward. Grasp a light dumbbell in each hand. Brace your torso by contracting your abdominal muscles. Slowly step forward with the right leg, placing your foot firmly on the ground. Keep your torso upright.

2. Inhale and bend your knees to lower your body toward the floor. Lunge only as far as you feel comfortable or your right thigh is parallel to the floor. Now, exhale and firmly push off with your right (front) leg and return to your starting position. Repeat with the left leg.

Note: This exercise can also be done without weights.

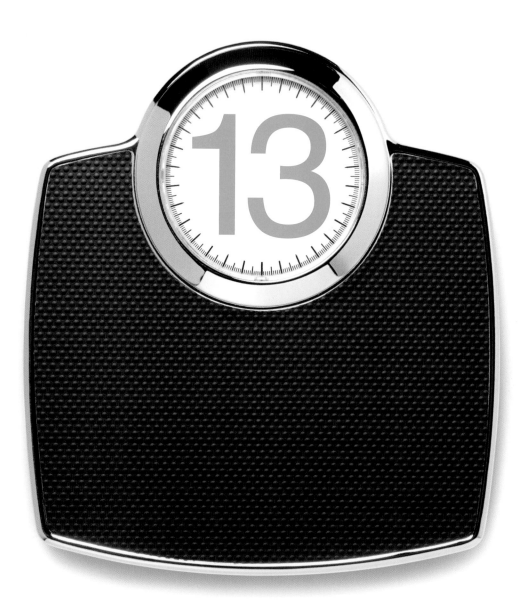

MAINTAIN YOUR GAINS
THE PALEO WAY

ONE OF THE MOST common downfalls of successful dieters is thinking that maintaining weight loss will draw on the same skills it took to lose the weight in the first place. Unfortunately, that's just not true. According to health statistics from the Centers for Disease Control and Prevention (CDC), only 20 percent of the people who go on a diet manage to maintain their weight loss for more than a year.

The trouble is that the skills we rely on to lose weight aren't all that useful when it comes to maintaining our weight loss. A 2011 national survey from researchers at universities around the United States—Penn State, Drexel, Ohio State, Stanford, and Texas—found several distinct strategies to losing weight, and they're different from the ones we need to keep the pounds off. Published in the *American Journal of Preventive Medicine,* the study suggests it's not simply a lack of willpower or self-control. Christopher Sciamanna, M.D., the study's lead author, queried 1,165 people about the behaviors they relied on to lose weight and, among those who were successful losers (they had kept off at least 10 percent of their weight for a year or more), how they had maintained that loss.

Sciamanna and his colleagues found that out of 36 specific practices used for short-term and long-term weight loss, 14 were specific to either the dieting phase or the maintenance phase, but not both. Yet these were the most valuable strategies, since they were most likely to predict success in either losing weight or keeping it off.

Nearly every study shows that weight loss peaks and regain starts at six months, points out Sciamanna, a professor of medicine and public health at Penn State College of Medicine. He's hopeful that the study findings can alter this pattern. While many of the key practices sound familiar, Sciamanna's research is the first to distinguish the role each plays in weight loss versus weight maintenance. Several of the strategies he looked at worked for both the active weight-loss phase and maintenance, and some of them will sound familiar to Paleo dieters. These are the behaviors you'll want to learn early and retain for the rest of your life:

- Eating plenty of lean sources of protein like fish, lean beef, and poultry
- Eating plenty of fruits and vegetables
- Limiting carbohydrates, especially junky ones such as chips and doughnuts
- Keeping careful control of portions
- Following a regular exercise routine
- Writing out—and sticking to—your grocery store list
- Paying attention to nutrition labels and avoiding processed foods

- Reminding and rewarding yourself for reaching and sustaining a healthy weight
- Weighing yourself regularly

Sciamanna's findings on weight-loss strategies can serve as a kind of road map to long-term success. But it's important to realize that you have to continue to pursue behaviors that will help you stay trim. Sciamanna points out that obesity is a chronic illness like hypertension; no one is surprised when a hypertensive patient stops taking their medication and their blood pressure rises, so it should be no surprise that when you stop using weight-control practices, the weight will come back all the same, he says.

We'll explore these valuable techniques and how they relate to your Paleo plan.

Keep Eating Paleo?

Once the weight comes off, you may be wondering whether you can or should continue to follow a Paleo plan. After all, you're omitting big food groups—do you need to abandon them for life?

You may not need to be quite as strict about your Paleo diet down the road—it all depends on how well the diet is working for you and how much you miss some of the foods you've given up. The decision is entirely up to you. If you're really craving a food you've eliminated—like bread, for example—try adding a serving or two a week to see how your body responds. Dying for some yogurt? Try it for breakfast on a Monday. But pay close attention to how your body responds: If you find that you're starving a couple of hours before lunchtime, it may not be the right food for maintaining your new figure.

If you decide to have a sandwich with whole wheat or sourdough bread, pay attention to how your stomach and digestive tract reacts over the next few hours. No problems? Good news—you can indulge in a sub every once in a while. However, if you feel bloated and your energy evaporates, you may want to stick with your Paleo alternatives to fill your sandwich cravings.

And if at any time your weight starts creeping up, you'll want to eliminate whatever non-Paleo food you've added back. The good news is that most people can manage a modified Paleo eating approach while preserving their weight loss. For the best results, try to stick with the Paleo basics 80-90 percent of the time to prevent occasional indulgences from sabotaging your success.

Keep Moving

If you're serious about avoiding regain, you'll need to stay active. One of the more robust research findings from the field of weight-loss maintenance has been the important role of regular exercise in keeping you slim. A study from the National Weight Control Registry found that people who were able to lose 30 pounds and keep it off for more than a year relied on a combination of diet and exercise; dieters who rely on one or the other aren't nearly as successful.

Lucky for you, you've already found the type of moves that keep you happy and engaged in staying fit; now you just have to be sure to make them a regular part of your life. That will mean staying injury free. One thing that will help is maintaining your strength, so continue to follow the strength-training regimen in Chaper 12. But you may also want to add a flexibility component to your exercise regimen. Regular stretching can keep your ligaments, tendons, and muscles pliable. A simple yoga routine can do wonders for your body, and it will help you release stress—which also plays a role in weight gain.

If you've never done yoga, check out a beginner's class in your area or try a DVD at home. You'll soon come to love the way regular stretching feels. It can feel like lubricating your joints—you'll move easier, your performance during exercise will improve, and you'll experience less soreness when you're finished. Just remember to start slowly, and go easy on your body. If you've never tried this type of stretching before, you may discover that your joints are nowhere near as flexible as the other participants in class or the instructor on your DVD. Don't worry about that, and definitely don't try to mimic or keep up with them. Listen to your body, and only bend as far as feels comfortable. With time, you'll become much more flexible (although some people never attain the flexibility on display in most yoga classes).

By the way, if you're looking for motivation to keep eating Paleo, a study from a couple of years ago shows that Paleo is well suited to your exercise efforts. Remember the old canard about carb-loading before you exert yourself? Turns out it isn't nearly as effective as protein-loading. Researchers at the University of Stirling in Scotland asked cyclists to follow two identical three-week training sessions. The first week was normal effort, the second week was intensified training, and the third week was a recovery period. During the first session, the cyclists consumed a high-protein diet (about 1.5 grams of protein per pound of body weight); during the second session they ate normal meals with normal protein content—about half that of the high-protein diet—and made up the difference with carbohydrates.

On the high-protein regimen, the athletes not only performed better, but they also recovered faster after the intense training sessions. The athletes also reported feeling stronger when they got more protein. In other words, to get the most out of your exercise—and to bring your best effort—eat Paleo.

Simple Portion Control

Take a look in your cupboard. Those Frisbee-sized dinner plates and helmet-sized cereal bowls aren't doing you or your family any favors. The sad truth is that we eat what's put in front of us, regardless how much there may be. Brian Wansink, a behavioral psychologist at Cornell University, has tested this in numerous ways.

(One of his most devious experiments was a soup bowl that could be filled surreptitiously from the bottom; sitting around a table, volunteers engaged in conversation would continue to eat as long as there was soup in the bowl, no matter how full they felt.) Wansink has found that reducing your plates by just 2 inches in diameter can reduce the amount of calories you take in by as much as 25 percent.

Choose smaller cereal bowls, and you'll get the same effect. Accounting for just breakfast and dinner, you could eliminate 350 calories a day. You could lose a pound every 10 days by doing this alone.

Shop Smart

As you have no doubt come to realize, a grocery list is invaluable when you're following a Paleo plan. To maintain your loss, you'll want to keep your kitchen well stocked with Paleo-friendly foods.

As you start experimenting with new Paleo-friendly foods, make sure you understand all the various labels on food packaging. Here's a quick guide:

"Fat-Free," "Low-Fat," "Reduced Fat," "Light"

When you see this on a package, it mostly means you can avoid it. You'll often see it on dairy products, though it turns up on almost every variety of food. These labels indicate a food has been processed, is no longer in its natural form, and doesn't belong in your Paleo diet. And there's little advantage to these claims on many foods: When fat is stripped away, food manufacturers usually increase the sugar and salt to make up for the lost flavor, which means you're getting just as many calories as you would with the regular food.

"Low Sodium," "Reduced Sodium"

"Low sodium" means the product has to deliver fewer than 140 milligrams per serving. But "reduced sodium" just means that you're getting 25 percent less salt than the original item. If a manufacturer is reducing the salt content of its food, it might be jacking up the sugar or fat content to boost flavor—compare the label to the original version.

"Contains Real Fruit"

Sadly, these labels rarely say how much real fruit the food contains. Even "100 percent real fruit juice" labels don't tell the whole story. These drinks are made from heavily processed and pasteurized juice concentrates, a process that wipes out plenty of nutrients and leaves plenty of sugar. The best way to get your fruit is in its original form. Skip the packaged stuff at the store.

Reward Yourself

Let's face it: You're putting a lot of hard work into losing weight and adapting to a new way of eating. So when you shed some pounds, indulge yourself: Shop for some new clothes or give yourself a night out at a Paleo-friendly restaurant. Maybe you need a tennis racquet, new exercise shoes, or a better bike. Set a weight goal and, when you hit it, give yourself a treat.

A Quick Restart

Anytime you regain weight, one of the first things you can try is restarting your food diary. This will help you track your Paleo versus non-Paleo food intake.

You may discover that you've let several less-than-nutritious foods creep back into your meals.

You may also discover that some new stress is pushing you to eat more, such as a new job, money pressures, or troubles with your kids. If emotions are driving you to overdo it, the quickest way to put your finger on the trouble, recognize it, and correct it is to use that food diary.

If things really get out of hand, try going through the four-week plan again. You'll quickly shed any pounds you may have regained, and you'll get a refresher course in Paleo eating.

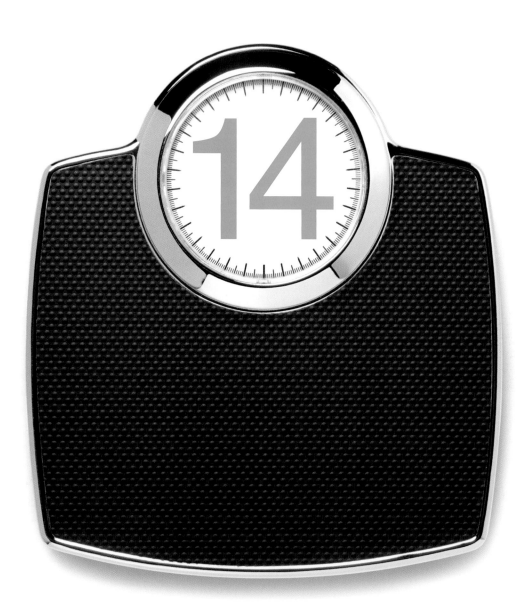

WHEN YOU'RE LOSING weight or trying to maintain your weight loss, you can't beat a little journaling to help you get a handle on the way you eat. A food diary is a powerful ally in your war on weight. Studies demonstrate that the food diary is a very consistent and reliable contributor to weight loss. Here are some tips for making a food journal work for you.

As it turns out, the simple act of writing down what you eat will make you more conscious of your intake and help you avoid overeating. Do it for the first four weeks of the diet, and you'll naturally become more conscious of your eating habits and choices.

Keeping a food diary can serve another purpose: Divining how much of your eating may be driven by your emotions. That's why there are entries for your mood on the diary pages that follow. Tracking when and why you eat may be as important to weight loss as tracking what you put on your plate. By cooking more and keeping Paleo food and snacks around the house, you can be sure that, when you eat, you'll choose food that will satisfy you and support your efforts to lose. But you'll also need to rein in urges to eat that are driven by stress, anger, loneliness, and other emotions.

For the next several weeks, keep the following diary pages with you. When you go to grab an unplanned bite to eat, record your emotional state. Are you bored? Are you upset about something that just happened? Are you mulling over a slight from earlier in the day? Then go ahead and eat, but halfway through, stop and make a note of how you're feeling after you've had some food.

After a week, flip back through the journal, and zero in on the times you saw a distinct improvement in your mood once you began eating. You've identified your emotional eating triggers, and now you can look for ways to replace the urge to eat with a healthier outlet for your feelings. A brisk walk, a phone call to a friend or loved one, or taking time for some deep breathing could make a big dent in your calorie intake. Perhaps one of the most interesting aspects of keeping a food journal while on a Paleo plan is that you'll find that you're thinking about eating much less than you once did. After a week or two, flip back through your journal, and note how your eating habits have changed!

DAY OF WEEK	TIME OF DAY	MEAL

What are you eating?	
How hungry are you?	
Where are you?	
Describe your mood.	

DAY OF WEEK	TIME OF DAY	MEAL

What are you eating?	
How hungry are you?	
Where are you?	
Describe your mood.	

DAY OF WEEK	TIME OF DAY	MEAL

What are you eating?	
How hungry are you?	
Where are you?	
Describe your mood.	

DAY OF WEEK	TIME OF DAY	MEAL

What are you eating?	
How hungry are you?	
Where are you?	
Describe your mood.	

DAY OF WEEK	TIME OF DAY	MEAL
What are you eating?		
How hungry are you?		
Where are you?		
Describe your mood.		

DAY OF WEEK	TIME OF DAY	MEAL
What are you eating?		
How hungry are you?		
Where are you?		
Describe your mood.		

DAY OF WEEK	TIME OF DAY	MEAL
What are you eating?		
How hungry are you?		
Where are you?		
Describe your mood.		

DAY OF WEEK	TIME OF DAY	MEAL
What are you eating?		
How hungry are you?		
Where are you?		
Describe your mood.		

DAY OF WEEK	TIME OF DAY	MEAL

What are you eating?	
How hungry are you?	
Where are you?	
Describe your mood.	

DAY OF WEEK	TIME OF DAY	MEAL

What are you eating?	
How hungry are you?	
Where are you?	
Describe your mood.	

DAY OF WEEK	TIME OF DAY	MEAL

What are you eating?	
How hungry are you?	
Where are you?	
Describe your mood.	

DAY OF WEEK	TIME OF DAY	MEAL

What are you eating?	
How hungry are you?	
Where are you?	
Describe your mood.	

DAY OF WEEK	TIME OF DAY	MEAL

What are you eating?	
How hungry are you?	
Where are you?	
Describe your mood.	

DAY OF WEEK	TIME OF DAY	MEAL

What are you eating?	
How hungry are you?	
Where are you?	
Describe your mood.	

DAY OF WEEK	TIME OF DAY	MEAL

What are you eating?	
How hungry are you?	
Where are you?	
Describe your mood.	

DAY OF WEEK	TIME OF DAY	MEAL

What are you eating?	
How hungry are you?	
Where are you?	
Describe your mood.	

DAY OF WEEK	TIME OF DAY	MEAL

What are you eating?	
How hungry are you?	
Where are you?	
Describe your mood.	

DAY OF WEEK	TIME OF DAY	MEAL

What are you eating?	
How hungry are you?	
Where are you?	
Describe your mood.	

DAY OF WEEK	TIME OF DAY	MEAL

What are you eating?	
How hungry are you?	
Where are you?	
Describe your mood.	

DAY OF WEEK	TIME OF DAY	MEAL

What are you eating?	
How hungry are you?	
Where are you?	
Describe your mood.	

DAY OF WEEK	TIME OF DAY	MEAL

What are you eating?	
How hungry are you?	
Where are you?	
Describe your mood.	

DAY OF WEEK	TIME OF DAY	MEAL

What are you eating?	
How hungry are you?	
Where are you?	
Describe your mood.	

DAY OF WEEK	TIME OF DAY	MEAL

What are you eating?	
How hungry are you?	
Where are you?	
Describe your mood.	

DAY OF WEEK	TIME OF DAY	MEAL

What are you eating?	
How hungry are you?	
Where are you?	
Describe your mood.	

DAY OF WEEK	TIME OF DAY	MEAL

What are you eating?	
How hungry are you?	
Where are you?	
Describe your mood.	

DAY OF WEEK	TIME OF DAY	MEAL

What are you eating?	
How hungry are you?	
Where are you?	
Describe your mood.	

DAY OF WEEK	TIME OF DAY	MEAL

What are you eating?	
How hungry are you?	
Where are you?	
Describe your mood.	

DAY OF WEEK	TIME OF DAY	MEAL

What are you eating?	
How hungry are you?	
Where are you?	
Describe your mood.	

Nutritional Information

HOW TO USE IT AND WHY

The following is a helpful guide to put the nutritional analysis numbers into perspective. Remember, one size doesn't fit all, so take your lifestyle, age, and circumstances into consideration when determining your nutrition needs.

IN OUR NUTRITIONAL ANALYSIS, WE USE THESE ABBREVIATIONS

sat saturated fat   **poly** polyunsaturated fat   **CHOL** cholesterol   **g** gram
mono monounsaturated fat   **CARB** carbohydrates   **CALC** calcium   **mg** milligram

DAILY NUTRITION GUIDE

	Women ages 25 to 50	Women over 50	Men ages 24 to 50	Men over 50
Calories	2,000	2,000 or less	2,700	2,500
Protein	50g	50g or less	63g	60g
Fat	65g or less	65g or less	88g or less	83g or less
Saturated Fat	20g or less	20g or less	27g or less	25g or less
Carbohydrates	304g	304g	410g	375g
Fiber	25g to 35g	25g to 35g	25g to 35g	25g to 35g
Cholesterol	300mg or less	300mg or less	300mg or less	300mg or less
Iron	18mg	8mg	8mg	8mg
Sodium	2,300mg or less	1,500mg or less	2,300mg or less	1,500mg or less
Calcium	1,000mg	1,200mg	1,000mg	1,000mg

The nutritional values used in our calculations either come from The Food Processor, Version 10.4 (ESHA Research), or are provided by food manufacturers.

Metric Equivalents

The information in the following charts is provided to help cooks outside the United States successfully use the recipes in this book. All equivalents are approximate.

COOKING/OVEN TEMPERATURE

Farenheit	225°F	250°F	275°F	300°F	325°F	350°F	375°F	400°F	425°F	450°F	475°F	500°F
Celsius	110°C	120°C	135°C	150°C	160°C	180°C	190°C	205°C	220°C	230°C	245°C	260°C

LENGTH
(To convert inches to centimeters, multiply the number of inches by 2.5.)

1 in =	2.5 cm
6 in = ½ ft =	15 cm
12 in = 1 ft =	30 cm
36 in = 3 ft = 1 yd =	90 cm
40 in =	100 cm = 1 m

LIQUID INGREDIENTS BY VOLUME

1 tsp =		1 ml
3 tsp = 1 Tbsp =	½ fl oz =	15 ml
2 Tbsp = ⅛ cup =	1 fl oz =	30 ml
16 Tbsp = 1 cup =	8 fl oz =	240 ml
1 pt = 2 cups =	16 fl oz =	480 ml
1 qt = 4 cups =	32 fl oz =	960 ml
	33 fl oz =	1000 ml = 1 l

DRY INGREDIENTS BY WEIGHT
(To convert ounces to grams, multiply the number of ounces by 30.)

1 oz = ¹⁄₁₆ lb =	30 g
4 oz = ¼ lb =	120 g
8 oz = ½ lb =	240 g
12 oz = ¾ lb =	360 g
16 oz = 1 lb =	480 g

References

Voegtlin, WL. *The Stone Age Diet*. New York: Vantage Press, Inc. 1975.

Eaton SB, Konner M. Paleolithic Nutrition: A consideration of its nature and current implications. *New England Journal of Medicine*. 1985; 312: 283-289.

Davis JL. The Risks of Belly Fat. WebMD. www.webmd.com

Atkinson SA, Josse AR, Phillips SM, Tarnopolsky MA. Increased consumption of dairy foods and protein during diet- and exercise-induced weight loss promotes fat mass and lean mass gain in overweight and obese premenopausal women. *Journal of Nutrition*. 2011; 141: 1626-1634.

Buendia JR, Bradlee ML, Singer MR, Moore LL. Diets Higher in Protein Predict Lower High Blood Pressure Risk in Framingham Offspring Study Adults. *American Journal of Hypertension*. 2014: hpu157v1-hpu157.

Dobrosielski D, Ouyang P, Shapiro E, Silber H, Stewart K, Zakaria S. Low-Carb, Higher-Fat Diets Add No Arterial Health Risks to Obese People Seeking to Lose Weight. John Hopkins Medicine. www.hopkinsmedicine.org

Centers for Disease Control and Prevention. Crude and Age-Adjusted Incidence of Diagnosed Diabetes per 1000 Population Aged 18-79 Years, United States, 1980-2011. www.cdc.gov

Sorensen LB, Soe M, Halkier KH, Stigsby B, Astrup A. Effects of increased dietary protein-to-carbohydrate rations in women with polycystic ovary syndrome. *The American Journal of Clinical Nutrition*. 2012; 95: 39-48.

Dietary Guidelines for Americans, 2010. www.dietaryguidelines.gov

Cordain L. *The Paleo Diet: Lose Weight and Get Healthy by Eating Foods You Were Designed to Eat*. New Jersey: John Wiley & Sons, Inc. 2002, 2011.

The Paleo Diet. www.thepaleodiet.com

Mark's Daily Apple. www.marksdailyapple.com

Astrup A, Dyerberg J, Elwood P, Hermansen K, Hu FB, Jakobsen MU, Kok FJ, Krauss RM, Lecerf JM, LeGrand P, Nestel P, Risérus U, Sanders T, Sinclair A, Stender S, Tholstrup T, Willet WC. The role of reducing intakes of saturated fat in prevention of cardiovascular disease; where does the evidence stand in 2010? *American Journal of Clinical Nutrition*. 2011; 93: 684-688.

Layman DK, Evans EM, Erickson D, Seyler J, Weber J, Bagshaw D, Griel A, Psota T, Kris-Etherton. A moderate-protein diet produces sustained weight loss and long-term changes in body composition and blood lipids in obese adults. *Journal of Nutrition*. 2009; 139: 514-521.

Boutcher SH. High-intensity exercise and fat loss. *Journal of Obesity*. 2011; 2011: 868305.

Trapp EG, Chisholm DJ, Freud J, Boutcher SH. The effects of high-intensity intermittent exercise training on fat loss and fasting insulin levels of young women. *International Journal of Obesity*. 2008; 32: 684-691.

For All-Day Metabolism Boost, Try Interval Training. American College of Sports Medicine. www.acsm.org

Wycherley TP, Noakes M, Clifton PM, Cleanthous X, Keogh JB, Brinkworth GD. High-Protein Diet with Resistance Exercise Training Improves Weight Loss and Body Composition in Overweight and Obese Patients with Type 2 Diabetes. *Diabetes Care*. 2010; 33: 969-976.

When to See a Doctor. American College of Sports Medicine. www.acsm.org

Physical Activity and Health. Centers for Disease Control and Prevention. www.cdc.gov

Sciamanna CN, Kiernan M, Rolls BJ, Boan J, Stuckey H, Kephart D, Miller CK. Practices Associated with Weight Loss Versus Weight-Loss Maintenance. *Preventative Medicine*. 2011; 41: 159-166.

Wansink B. Why Visual Cues of Portion Size May Influence Intake. Cornell University Food and Brand Lab. www.foodpsychology.cornell.edu

Index

ISBN-13: 978-0-8487-4452-6
ISBN-10: 0-8487-4452-7
Library of Congress Control Number: 2015933189

Printed in the United States of America
First Printing 2015

Be sure to check with your health-care provider
before making any changes in your diet.

Oxmoor House
Editorial Director: Anja Schmidt
Creative Director: Felicity Keane
Art Director: Christopher Rhoads
Executive Photography Director: Iain Bagwell
Executive Food Director: Grace Parisi
Photo Editor: Kellie Lindsey
Managing Editor: Elizabeth Tyler Austin
Assistant Managing Editor: Jeanne de Lathouder

The 10 Pounds Off Paleo Diet
Senior Editor: Andrea C. Kirkland, M.S., R.D.
Editorial Assistant: April Smitherman
Assistant Test Kitchen Manager:
   Alyson Moreland Haynes
Recipe Developers and Testers: Julia Levy
   Stefanie Maloney, Callie Nash, Karen Rankin
Food Stylists: Nathan Carrabba,
   Victoria E. Cox, Margaret Monroe Dickey,
   Catherine Crowell Steele
Senior Photographer: Hélène Dujardin

Senior Photo Stylists: Kay E. Clarke,
   Mindi Shapiro Levine
Senior Production Manager: Greg A. Amason
Assistant Production Director: Sue Chodakiewicz

Contributors
Writer: John Hastings
Assistant Project Editor: Melissa Brown
Designer: Ben Margherita
Junior Designer: AnnaMaria Jacob
Compositor: Anna Ramia
Copy Editors: Dolores Hydock,
   *Marra*thon Production Services
Proofreaders: Julie Bosche,
   Norma Butterworth-McKittrick,
Indexer: *Marra*thon Production Services
Nutrition Reviewer: Amy Kubal, R.D.
Fitness Reviewer: Michele Stanten
Fellows: Laura Arnold, Kylie Dazzo, Nicole Fisher,
   Loren Lorenzo, Caroline Smith, Amanda Widis
Photographer: Stephen DeVries
Photo Stylist: Missie Crawford

Time Inc. Books
Publisher: Margot Schupf
Vice President, Finance: Vandana Patel
Executive Director, Marketing Services:
   Carol Pittard
Executive Director, Business Development:
   Suzanne Albert
Executive Director, Marketing: Susan Hettleman
Assistant General Counsel: Simone Procas
Assistant Project Manager: Allyson Angle

Photo Credits
Courtesy of: 17 Sarah Livingston, before and
after; 29 Bob Montgomery, before and after; 41
Chae Fields, before and after **Getty Images:**
6, 10, 20, 28, 42, 50, 62, 66, 86, 106, 144, 164, 188,
202, 210 DNY59, scale; 34 Jason Loucas, hamburger buns; 39 Diane Macdonald, carrot sticks

Back Cover
Seared Steak Salad, page 103